EUCAMBIS: IMMUNOLOGY AND AGEING IN EUROPE

Biomedical and Health Research

Volume 29

Earlier published in this series

Vol. 1. G.N. Fracchia and M. Theofilatou (Eds.), Health Services Research
Vol. 2. J.E.W. Beneken and V. Thévenin (Eds.), Advances in Biomedical Engineering
Vol. 3. C. Baya † (Ed.), Advances in Medical Biology
Vol. 4. K. Vuylsteek and M. Hallen (Eds.), Epidemiology
Vol. 5. A.J.M. Vermorken and F.A.J.M. Schermer (Eds.), Towards Coordination of Cancer Research in Europe
Vol. 6. A.-E. Baert, M.A. Koch, L. Montagnier, M.C. Razquin and D. Tyrrell (Eds.), AIDS Research at EC Level
Vol. 7. G.N. Fracchia (Ed.), European Medicines Research
Vol. 8. M. Hallen and A. Klepsch (Eds.), Human Genome Analysis Programme
Vol. 9. A.-E. Baert, S.S. Baig, C. Bardoux, G.N. Fracchia, M. Hallen, O. Le Dour, M.C. Razquin, V. Thévenin, A. Vanvossel and M. Vidal (Eds.), European Union Biomedical and Health Research
Vol. 10. F.F. Cruz-Sánchez, R. Ravid and M.L. Cuzner (Eds.), Neuropathological Diagnostic Criteria for Brain Banking
Vol. 11. S.S. Baig (Ed.), Cancer Research at the European Level
Vol. 12. M. Maio (Ed.), Immunology of Human Melanoma
Vol. 13. V.K. Hopsu-Havu, M. Järvinen and H. Kirschke (Eds.), Proteolysis in Cell Functions
Vol. 14. G. ter Heege (Ed.), EURO-QUAL
Vol. 15. N. Katunuma, H. Kido, H. Fritz and J. Travis (Eds.), Medical Aspects of Proteases and Protease Inhibitors
Vol. 16. P.I. Haris and D. Chapman (Eds.), New Biomedical Materials
Vol. 17. J.J.F. Schroots, R. Fernandez-Ballesteros and G. Rudinger (Eds.), Aging in Europe
Vol. 18. R. Leidl (Ed.), Health Care and its Financing in the Single European Market
Vol. 19. P. Jenner and R. Demirdamar (Eds.), Dopamine Receptor Subtypes
Vol. 20. P.I. Haris and D. Chapman (Eds.), Biomembrane Structures
Vol. 21. N. Yoganandan, F.A. Pintar, S.J. Larson and A. Sances Jr. (Eds.), Frontiers in Head and Neck Trauma
Vol. 22. J. Matsoukas and T. Mavromoustakos (Eds.), Bioactive Peptides in Drug Discovery and Design: Medical Aspects
Vol. 23. M. Hallen (Ed.), Human Genome Analysis
Vol. 24. S.S. Baig (Ed.), Cancer Research Supported under BIOMED 1
Vol. 25. N.J. Gooderham (Ed.), Drug Metabolism: Towards the Next Millennium
Vol. 26. P. Jenner (Ed.), A Molecular Biology Approach to Parkinson's Disease
Vol. 27. P.A. Frey and D.B. Northrop (Eds.), Enzymatic Mechanisms
Vol. 28. A.M.N. Gardner and R. Fox, The Venous System in Health and Disease

ISSN: 0929-6743

EUCAMBIS: Immunology and Ageing in Europe

Edited by

G. Pawelec

Tübingen Ageing and Tumor Immunology Group,
Section of Transplantation Immunology, Tübingen, Germany

IOS Press

Ohmsha

Amsterdam • Berlin • Oxford • Tokyo • Washington, DC

ISBN 90 5199 434 6 (IOS Press)
ISBN 4 274 90317 6 C3047 (Ohmsha)
Library of Congress Catalog Card Number: 99-68067

Publisher
IOS Press
Van Diemenstraat 94
1013 CN Amsterdam
The Netherlands
fax: +31 20 620 3419
e-mail: order@iospress.nl

Distributor in the UK and Ireland
IOS Press/Lavis Marketing
73 Lime Walk
Headington
Oxford OX3 7AD
England
fax: +44 1865 75 0079

Distributor in the USA and Canada
IOS Press, Inc.
5795-G Burke Centre Parkway
Burke, VA 22015
USA
fax: +1 703 323 3668
e-mail: iosbooks@iospress.com

Distributor in Germany
IOS Press
Spandauer Strasse 2
D-10178 Berlin
Germany
fax: +49 30 242 3113

Distributor in Japan
Ohmsha, Ltd.
3-1 Kanda Nishiki-cho
Chiyoda-ku, Tokyo 101
Japan
fax: +81 3 3233 2426

Cover illustration: picture of a chromosome spread with telomeres lit up. Thanks to DAKO GmbH, Hamburg, Germany for permission to use this picture.

PRINTED IN THE NETHERLANDS

Contents

The European Union Concerted Action on the Molecular Biology of Immunosenescence (EUCAMBIS)

Graham PAWELEC
Tübingen Ageing and Tumour Immunology (TATI) Group, Section for Transplantation Immunology and Immunohaematology, Center for Medical Research of the University of Tübingen (ZMF), Waldhörnlestr. 22, D-72072 Tübingen, Germany

Abstract: EUCAMBIS was established under BIOMED I from 1994 to 1998 as an interdisciplinary consortium aiming to advance our understanding of the molecular and cellular bases of immunosenescence. The project sought to draw together scientists and clinicians from diverse fields including immunology, molecular biology, cell and tumour biology, geriatrics, endocrinology, rheumatology and transplantation biology in order to investigate the impact of ageing on immune responses. The papers collected in this volume illustrate the diversity of some of the work carried out by associates of EUCAMBIS during its three-and-a-half year existence. This introductory chapter attempts to summarize the results of some of the EUCAMBIS collaborations, with emphasis on a workshop approach which was aimed at analysing the expression of genes contributing to growth arrest in ageing human T lymphocytes.

1. Research Activities of the EUCAMBIS Participants

There is increasingly good evidence that immunosenescence is clinically relevant for protection against infectious disease in the elderly. Many major causes of death show deceleration or neutrality with increasing age in the very old, whereas those which continue to accelerate mostly involve infectious agents, ie. pneumonia, influenza, gastroenteritis, bronchitis (Horiuchi and Wilmoth, J. Gerontol. Ser. A-Biol. Sci. Med. 52, B67-B77, 1997). This suggests that failing immunity results in increased incidence of those diseases that the immune system is designed to protect against, ie. infectious diseases. EUCAMBIS-member E. Remarque (Leiden) continues to work intensively in this area, particularly in the efficacy of influenza vaccination in the elderly and prediction of infectious disease morbidity by means of immunogerontological biomarkers. From longitudinal studies, it may become possible to identify individuals with an immunological "risk" phenotype (Wikby et al., Mech. Ageing. Dev. 102, 187-198, 1998); thus far, however, there are no data on cause of death of the persons with such risk phenotypes or with measured immunological parameters interpreted as dysfunctional. This is a difficult problem because, amongst other reasons, even the cause of death may be hard to establish unequivocally in the elderly. E. Remarque is also currently investigating diagnoses at hospital admission in the Leiden over-85 study in order to try to shed some light on this.

These findings of course again pose the question of whether the alterations that can be observed in the immune parameters of the elderly are a cause or a result of underlying disease processes. For this reason, much attention has been paid in human immunogerontology to the question of donor selection. Procedures for screening health status have been developed, with the "SENIEUR" protocol gaining the most widespread acceptance. Alterations to the SENIEUR protocol by its originator, EUCAMBIS-member G. Ligthart (Amsterdam), are continuing. The original SENIEUR protocol is a very strict protocol based primarily on objective laboratory values but which excludes the great majority even of apparently healthy old donors (and one third of young donors as well - although this reduces to 10% if alterations in laboratory values due to use of oral contraceptives are excluded). However, the use of SENIEUR donors may come closer to realizing the ambition of separating underlying disease from intrinsic ageing processes in assessing age-associated effects on the immune system. It is becoming clearer from several studies that donors who do have SENIEUR status do behave differently in tests of immune function compared to non-SENIEUR donors, although they also show alterations in immune function compared to young donors selected according to the same criteria. It would be desirable to perform longitudinal studies with SENIEUR donors and to assess whether loss of SENIEUR status correlates with altered immunological parameters and increased mortality. These studies are in practise very difficult to carry out. However, preliminary data on the association between loss of SENIEUR status and poorer prognosis have been forthcoming. E. Remarque is currently evaluating the results of a three-year follow-up on this.

Other data illustrating the importance of the immune system in healthy ageing come from studies on centenarians. By and large, unlike the "average" younger elderly, healthy centenarians are found to have well-preserved immune functions, much more similar to the "young" immune system. Two EUCAMBIS members, E. Mariani (Bologna) and R. Solana (Cordóba) have recently made some inroads in the study of immunosenescence in centenarians with emphasis on alterations in NK activity, which may possibly be equally or even more important than changes in T cell status.

Longitudinal studies themselves, even if performed with stringently selected donors still cannot demonstrate that measured parameters which are predictive of an outcome are actually causally related to that outcome. One possibility to approach this question is to test interventions which seek to redress a balance perceived to be suboptimal in the aged compared to the young. However, direct interventions to "boost" the aged immune system have been undertaken according to accepted scientific method in humans only as far as correcting nutritional deficiencies is concerned. These trials have been based on supplementation of micronutrients and vitamins in the elderly, who are commonly malnourished in this and other respects. Varying degrees of success have been reported but such trials still do not address the question of the ageing immune system *per se*. EUCAMBIS member Y. Barnett (Coleraine) is involved in such supplementation trials at the University of Ulster, measuring mutation rates in human T cells and assessing the effect of dietary anti-oxidant vitamin supplementation on these.

The main strategy for life extension in rodents, namely caloric restriction, has not been definitively demonstrated to be effective in primates, let alone humans, and the few individuals attempting to practise this regime are not participating in any controlled trials. Another type of manipulation which seems very successful at improving the immune function of aged rodents, ie. hormone replacement or supplementation, has also yielded unconvincing results in man. Melatonin supplementation has been utilized by the general public in an uncontrolled fashion with dubious and unproven benefits; dehydroepiandrosterone replacement therapy has at least been tested properly in some trials, but with negative results. A relatively new direction which will be taken in immunosenescence studies must be to attempt to unravel the neuroendocrinological and other hormonal effects on immune responsiveness in ageing. Here, EUCAMBIS-member C. Bartoloni (Rome), working together with G. Doria and D. Frasca in Rome, and R. Solana working together with M. de la Fuente (Madrid) are actively exploring such interactions at the T cell level.

Today, immunogerontology stands at a crossroads where it is critical to demonstrate its clinical relevance once and for all. The belief that age-associated changes in immunity must impact on the individual´s health and well-being is firmly ensconced but on close examination not actually proven. Nonetheless, improved comprehension of the details of age-associated changes in man is critical for understanding the results of intervention trials and designing more rational approaches. Because the immune response is guided by T cells which must undergo extensive clonal proliferation on contact with antigen in primary responses and repeated clonal expansion for memory responses, EUCAMBIS concentrates on T cells. Replicative senescence may be particularly important for T cell responses as reviewed recently by several EUCAMBIS members (eg. see ref. (Pawelec et al., Frontiers in Biosciences. 4, d216 (www.bioscience.org), 1999). Proliferative lifespans and replicative senescence have been extensively studied in other tissues, particularly fibroblasts, but relatively little is known about the behaviour of T cells in this context and the molecular biology of their growth control. To this end, EUCAMBIS members S. Shall (Brighton), C. Paraskeva (Bristol) and G. Pawelec (Tübingen) have examined the control of lymphocyte proliferation, costimulation, apoptosis induction and memory cell maintenance in vitro using cultured human T cells in comparison to other cells such as normal and Werner´s Syndrome fibroblasts (standard senescence model excluding apoptosis) or colon cells (model for rapid proliferation terminating in apoptosis). T cell clones in vitro provide a model to study "longitudinal" age-associated changes during extended culture. G. Pawelec focussed on CD4+ Th0-type cells derived from normal CD3+ adult peripheral T cells, or extrathymically from CD3- adult bone marrow cells (pre-T cells), or more recently from CD34+ "stem" cells. These clones have finite lifespans and show some alterations in surface molecules which may contribute to their observed altered responsiveness to activation signals during progression through their lifespan. They may provide a useful model for studying the effects of "clonal exhaustion" at the cell molecular biological levels. Molecular biological investigations have centered around growth control by TGF-ß-sensitive gene programs by V. Sorrentino (Milan) and mitotic inhibitors spontaneously activated in old cells (Pawelec) as well as searching for novel genes in these two systems (Sorrentino, Pawelec). We have demonstrated enhanced expression of the IL 2 transcription repressor NiIL2a and decreased expression of the NF-ATp transcription factor in senescent compared to young T cell clones, and increased expression of the mitotic inhibitor p27. Our search for novel genes has progressed to the point where we have a number of partially sequenced candidates but still no unequivocally identified genes which are universally upregulated in senescent T cells.

Data such as these may be relevant not only for studies of immunosenescence in the elderly, but particularly for studying ageing of the immune response in younger individuals as well, for example, during chronic infections or other chronic disease states, such as leukemias (the area in which EUCAMBIS member G.M. Taylor (Manchester) is active) and possibly also in non-physiological situations of chronic antigenic stimulation such as in organ transplantation (B. Bradley, Bristol). Finally, the dysregulation of clonal expansion, apoptosis and memory cell formation may be of tremendous importance in autoimmune disease. Understanding the pathological characteristics of rheumatoid arthritis may be extremely informative about the regular processes of T cell differentiation and control of the normal T cell response (M. Salmon, Birmingham and A. Akbar, London).

2. The EUCAMBIS Workshop

Thus, deterioration of the immune system with aging ("immunosenescence") is believed to contribute to morbidity and mortality in man due to the greater incidence of infection, as well as possibly autoimmune phenomena and cancer in the aged. Dysregulation of T cell function is thought to play a critical part in these processes. Factors contributing to T cell immunosenescence may include a) stem cell defects, b) thymus involution, c) defects in antigen presenting cells, d) aging of resting immune cells, e) disrupted activation pathways in immune cells, f) replicative senescence of clonally expanding cells. Moreover, T cell replicative senescence may represent a form of ageing of critical importance for immunity in young individuals as well as in the aged, eg. in cases of chronic antigenic stimulation. For this reason, studies of T cell replicative senescence may be of relevance to infectious disease, cancer and organ transplantation, and not only to geriatrics.

The participants of EUCAMBIS included investigators working in all of these areas, but it was particularly the latter point, replicative senescence, which occupied center stage in the "workshop" collaboration for the reason mentioned above. This workshop was aimed at identifying genes which are upregulated during ageing, 1) initially by using substractive hybridisation techniques, later by differential display methodology, with old and young cells from the same clonal populations, and 2) by screening for the expression of known genes available from other laboratories.

3. Progress report on the EUCAMBIS workshop "Expression of cell-cycle control / growth arrest genes in young and old T cells"

The participants received PCR primers for actin, IL 2, $p16^{Ink4}$, $p21^{sdi}$ and $p27^{kip1}$ to analyse in semi-quantitative assays mRNA expression in T cells and/or NK cells from young and old donors or cultured cell clones. The primers were synthesized in large amounts by one company and the same well-characterized batch shipped to the participants.

1) the results of the semi-quantitative PCR experiments performed in participants' laboratories and repeated on the same materials in the central facility in Tübingen were only poorly reproducible (68% agreement). And this although we had tried hard to standardize all possible factors. A preliminary conclusion would therefore be that it is very hard to compare results using this method between different laboratories, even 'though we tried to keep the system as simple as possible;

2) so far there is little evidence for any consistent difference in the level of expression of mRNA for p16, p21 and p27 in resting or stimulated PBMC from SENIEUR donors compared with JUNIEUR donors (Table 1).

Results shown in Table 1 indicate that the expression of the selected control gene, ß-actin, is similar in cells from young and old donors, because mRNA became detectable in all cases after 23 PCR cycles, regardless of whether they were stimulated or not. No IL 2 message was detectable in SENIEUR donors' PBMC, but became detectable after 27 cycles on stimulation. JUNIEUR donors' PBMC, on the other hand, did contain IL 2 message, but this was present in higher amounts after stimulation (ie. became visible after 24 PCR cycles in stimulated cells as compared to 28 cycles in resting cells). However, for both p21 and p27 message, there appeared to be more present in JUNIEUR cells, whereas p16 message was essentially undetectable in any of the cells.

Table 1 **Mitotic inhibitor mRNA in PBMC**

	p16	p21	p27	ß-actin	IL 2
SENIEUR, resting	∞	28	30	23	∞
SENIEUR, stimulated	35	27	28	23	27
JUNIEUR, resting	∞	27	29	23	28
JUNIEUR, stimulated	∞	23	26	23	24

n = 5 in each group, resting = cryopreserved PBMC ex-vivo; stimulated = PHA-activated for 2 days

However, in the case of T cell clones, there may be significant differences which need to be followed up and confirmed (Table 2). Thus, it seemed fairly clear that p16 mRNA was expressed in the cloned cells and to a greater extent in the old cells. The same was even more strikingly true for p21, which was not detectable in young cells, but present at the same level as actin in the old cells. Expression of p27 was also greater in the old cells, whereas ß-actin message levels werre identical in young and old cells. The picture here may be much clearer because of the use of well-defined homogeneous, albeit strongly selected, clonal populations for these assays.

Table 2 **Mitotic inhibitor mRNA in T cell clones**

Clones	p16	p21	p27	ß-actin
Old, resting	23	23	25	23
Old, stimulated	23	23	25	23
Young, resting	27	∞	29	23
Young, stimulated	27	∞	29	23

Young = <35 PD, old = > 43 PD, n = 5 CD4+ TCC, tested pairwise. Data represent mean number of PCR cycles at which bands became visible. Resting = 14 days after stimulation; stimulated = 6 hours after immobilized CD3 mAb + IL 2

4. Future perspectives

The interactions and collaborations established between the founding members of EUCAMBIS and extended by addition of further associates during the existence of the project have been to a great extent continued to the present time. The central cell and data bank established by EUCAMBIS (with the generous additional support of the Messer-Griesheim Company) is being maintained and expanded. The EUCAMBIS web-site is also still maintained (www.medizin.uni-tuebingen.de/eucambis/). The Fifth Framework Program of the European Commission saw the creation of a special "Key Action" on "Ageing and Disabilities" aimed at networking diverse European research in this area and focussing on matters of practical relevance to the well-being of the European Community. This objective is to be lauded provided that the essential contribution of basic research is not undervalued. To this end, EUCAMBIS strives to transform itself into a larger "thematic network" of groups including several of the founder members, but with many additional investigators as well. Our aim will be to exploit the longitudinal culture model of human T cell clones using a wide range of investigatory techniques to pinpoint alterations in T cells which contribute causally and critically to the ageing process in vitro. These candidates will then be validated on ex vivo cells from healthy and less healthy young and old donors, centenarians, progeria patients, persons participating in longitudinal ageing studies as well as dietary intervention trials and vaccination trials. In addition, T cells from sources of chronic antigen exposure including those infiltrating tumours, transplanted organs and rheumatoid synovium will be studied. This type of "workshop" approach will again tie the participants together in a joint action; at the same time, the thematic network will provide an "umbrella" under which each participant will attempt to cluster their own research projects together with other members of the thematic network and outside scientists in order to present a coherent group of projects to the Commission for coordinated support.

5. Acknowledgements

First and foremost, we are grateful for the financial support for this project (BMHI-CT94-1209) from the EC and to the help and encouragement from the DG12 Scientific Officers at all times. In addition, many companies contributed to supporting this work, most frequently in the form of sponsoring meetings. We are particularly indebted to the Messer-Griesheim Company for making liquid nitrogen storage and handling facilities available for the cell bank in the Central Facility in Tübingen. Support for the work in the Coordinator's laboratory, which contributed materially to the success of the EUCAMBIS project, came from the Deutsche Forschungsgemeinschaft, the Mildred Scheel Foundation, The VERUM Foundation and the Sandoz Foundation for Gerontological Research. We would like also to thank the then-Editor-in-Chief (Prof. B. Strehler) and the publishers of "Mechanisms of Ageing and Development" for their help and encouragement in publishing EUCAMBIS-related material, and to "Immunology Today" for publishing EUCAMBIS meeting summaries. There follows a list of such publications relating to joint EUCAMBIS reports, meeting reports and position papers.

6. EUCAMBIS-related publications

Pawelec G: Molecular and cell biological studies of ageing and their application to considerations of T lymphocyte immunosenescence. Mech Ageing Dev 79:1 (1995).

Pawelec G, Adibzadeh M, Pohla H, Schaudt K: Immunosenescence: ageing of the immune system. Immunol Today 16:420, 1995.

Pawelec G, Sansom D, Rehbein A, Adibzadeh M, Beckmann I: Decreased proliferative capacity and increased susceptibility to activation-induced cells death in late-passage human CD4+ TCR2+ cultured T cell clones. Exp Gerontol 31:655, 1996.

Adibzadeh M, Mariani E, Bartoloni C, Beckman I, Ligthart G, Remarque E, Shall S, Solana R, Taylor GM, Barnett Y, Pawelec G: Lifespans of T lymphocytes. Mech Ageing Dev 91:145, 1996.

Pawelec G, Adibzadeh M, Solana R, Beckman I: The T cell in the ageing individual (lecture from the First International Conference on Ageing and Immunology, Washington DC, June 1996). Mech Ageing Dev 93:35, 1997

Effros R, Pawelec G: Replicative senescence of T lymphocytes: does the Hayflick Limit lead to immune exhaustion? Immunol Today 18:450, 1997.

Pawelec G, Mariani E, Offringa R, Melief CJM, Solana R: Generation and characterization of killer cells. In: Immunological Methods in Microbiology (eds. SHE Kaufmann, D Kabelitz), series "Methods in Microbiology", Academic Press, London, pp. 605-619, 1998.

Remarque E, Pawelec G: T cell immunosenescence and its clinical relevance in man. Rev Clin Gerontol 8:5, 1998.

Pawelec G, Rehbein A, Haehnel K, Merl A, Adibzadeh M: Human T cell clones in long-term culture as a model of immunosenescence. Immunol. Rev. 160:31, 1997.

Pawelec G, Solana R: Immunosenescence. Immunol Today 18:514, 1997.

Pawelec G, Y. Barnett, Solana R, Remarque E: T cell immunosenescence. Frontiers in Bioscience 3:59-99, 1998 (access via http://www.bioscience.org)

Solana R, Pawelec G: Molecular and Cellular Basis of Immunosenescence (Preface to a Special Issue, Proceedings of the 5th EUCAMBIS meeting). Mech Ageing Dev 102:115, 1998.

Pawelec G, Solana R, Remarque E, Mariani E: Impact of aging on innate immunity in man. J Leuk Biol 64:703, 1998.

Pawelec G: T cell clones. In: Methods in Molecular Medicine: Aging Methods and Protocols (Eds. C. Barnett & Y. Barnett), Humana Press (in press).

Engel A, Adibzadeh M, Pawelec G: DDRT-PCR. In: Methods in Molecular Medicine: Aging Methods and Protocols (Eds. C. Barnett & Y. Barnett), Humana Press (in press).

Pawelec G. Immunosenescence: impact in the young as well as the old? Mech Ageing Dev 108:1, 1999.

Pawelec G, Effros RB, Caruso C, Remarque E, Barnett Y, Solana R: T cells and aging. Frontiers in Bioscience 4:d216, 1999 (access via http://www.bioscience.org)

Pawelec G: Importance of immunosenescence for adoptive immunotherapy of cancer in humans? J Anti-Aging Med (in press).

EUCAMBIS: Immunology and Ageing in Europe
G. Pawelec (Ed.)
IOS Press, 2000

Human T cell clones as tools to study immunosenescence

Graham PAWELEC, Medi ADIBZADEH, Wolfgang WAGNER and Andrea ENGEL
Tübingen Ageing and Tumour Immunology (TATI) Group, Section for Transplantation Immunology and Immunohaematology, Center for Medical Research of the University of Tübingen (ZMF), Waldhörnlestr. 22, D-72072 Tübingen, Germany

Abstract. Like other normal somatic tissue cells, human T lymphocytes have finite lifespans in vitro. For CD4+ helper cells this averages around 35 population doublings (PD) for established T cell clones (TCC) derived from mature peripheral T cells of young adults, but only around an estimated 17 PD for the entire population. However, a minority of clones experience lifespans of at least twice the average and in rare cases, much more (up to 150 PD). TCC derived from CD34+ stem cells in vitro have similar lifespans, suggesting that "ageing" of the cells begins after their maturation into T cells in vitro. Similarly and perhaps at first sight surprisingly, T cells from perfectly healthy (SENIEUR) nonagenarians can be cloned at the same level of efficiency and with a similar longevity as those from the young. Longitudinal studies of T cells from these different sources ageing in vitro reveal candidate functional and structural characteristics which may correlate with the ageing process and which can be validated ex vivo on freshly isolated T cells from the elderly. The challenge for the future remains to delineate which of these candidate factors is causally related to T cell ageing and to discover means to prevent or reverse this.

1. Introduction

Immunosenescence is here taken to mean the dysregulation and deterioration of immune function in the elderly, and believed to cause an increased susceptibility to infectious diseases and perhaps other diseases of the aged. Specific acquired immune responses are the responsibility of T cells and B cells. The latter depend on the appropriate function of the T cell system, which in turn depends upon intact innate immunity. Ageing does affect the innate immune system in many ways [1] but antigen presentation seems to be remarkably well-preserved in the elderly [2]. After activation by antigen, the immune response depends on the clonal expansion of relatively small numbers of T cell clones, each to sufficient numbers for effective immunity. Given a precursor frequency for antigen-specific T cells of around 1 in 10,000 - 100,000, and a clone size of 10^8 or more during acute infection [3], around 28 PD may be required of each TCC. After completion of the response, 99% of the cells may die by apoptosis and the survivors become memory cells [4].

Rechallenge during a later infection would cause these memory cells again to divide to generate sufficient cells for a secondary response. Given the finite lifespans of somatic cells, such extensive clonal expansion might confront the responding T cells with clonal exhaustion [5]. In order to investigate T cell ageing in a model system, and to quantitate precisely the average and maximum lifespans of human T lymphocytes, we have concentrated in our own laboratory and as part of the EUCAMBIS collaboration on studying monoclonal populations. This is necessary because in clonal populations (and only in clonal populations) is it possible to follow longitudinally the behaviour of a single cell line with certainty that changes observed are not due to alterations in the proportions of the different cell types present. In addition, although at first sight paradoxical, the calculation of longevities of mixed populations can only be done by looking at each component clone separately. If this is not taken into account, only the longevity of the longest surviving clone from the original polyclonal population can be assessed. This is one of the confounding factors even in investigations of a much more extensively studied cell type, the fibroblast, where almost all available data actually apply only to the longest-lived clone present, and not to the average longevity of the entire population. In fact, it is one of the reasons for recent misconceived arguments in the literature concerning the validity and in vivo relevance of the so-called "Hayflick Limit" to the proliferation of cells in culture and the controversy over whether cells taken from elderly individuals have a lesser remaining proliferative capacity than those from the young [6]. Regarding human T cells in the context of this controversy, the one publication in the literature in the past which examined this question concluded from data on lifespans of *whole* T cell populations that there was no correlation between the age of the donor and lifespan of the culture. However, at the *clonal* level, on the basis of rather few data, these authors did in fact find such a correlation [7]. To redress this imbalance, we have (over the years) attempted to culture all derived clones from at least some experiments to the end of their finite lifespans. Moreover, we have attempted to compare average and maximum longevities of clones from different sources: mature $CD3^+$ T cells from young donors or healthy old donors, as well as from patients with certain diseases (the latter not included in the present analysis), compared to extra-thymically differentiated T cells derived from either CD3-negative $CD7^+$ progenitors of $CD34^+$ stem cells.

2. Longevities of TCC from young donors

Table 1 shows a summary of the cloning efficiencies (CE) and longevities of TCC derived from these different sources and cultured under different conditions. T cells were alloactivated and cloned by limiting dilution in the presence of a pool of irradiated PBMC from numerous donors, in medium supplemented with 20 U/ml purified natural IL 2 and 10% human serum [8]. This represents the standard cloning procedure applied in the first experiments (labelled CD3, young, HS in the Table). Growing clones were transferred from 1 mm-diameter culture wells to 7 mm after 6 - 10 days and thereafter to 16 mm wells in which they were maintained. Cloning efficiency was calculated from values obtained by scoring positive those 1 mm-diameter wells which were at least one-third full. This represents ca. 1000 T cells, which is equivalent to about 10 population doublings (PD). No attempt has been made to assess the number of cell divisions undergone in each clone, but if none of the progeny of each division dies, this is equivalent to the PD undergone. Ages of clones are therefore always expressed in PD, but this is clearly an underestimate of cell divisions because not all progeny of each division do survive, especially as the clones age. Estimation of the number of PD undergone itself requires the acceptance of further approximations. First, because cloning efficiency was defined as including only those cells capable of at least 10 PD, any cells generating less than 10 PD were excluded from the calculations of average population longevity, ie, only T cells which were defined as clonable by our arbitrary criteria were taken into account in this assessment. Cells transferred from 1 mm to 7 mm-diameter wells were scored positive, but not all of them continued to grow in the larger wells. Those that grew and were transferred numbered ca. 1 x 10^5 (equivalent to about 17 PD) and this was used as the basis for calculating their longevity in PD. However, those that did not survive may have managed anything from the original 10 PD to 17 PD. It was therefore decided to consider that those clones dying off between transfers had in fact undergone 17 PD and this figure was used to calculate average longevity of all derived clones. After the cells were transferred to 16 mm-diameter they were assessed for the actual number of PD undergone. As can be seen from Table 1, $CD3^+$ cells from normal healthy young adult donors commonly yield average CE of around 50%. However, only about half of these clones reach a population size of one million (equivalent to 20 PD). TCC continue to be lost thereafter so that there are fewer and fewer survivors at 30 and 40 PD. The average longevity of the established clones (ie. taken as those that reach 20 PD) in these experiments comes to approximately 33 PD, whereas the average lifespan of all cells in the starting population is considerably less, being estimated at only approximately 17 PD. This contrasts very markedly with the lifespan of the longest-lived clone in any of these experiments, which was around 170 PD. This represents a truly astronomical number of cells, around 10^{51}. Clearly, rare long-lived clones are the exception rather than the rule for these cultures. This implies that if similar phenomena occur in vivo, these longest-lived clones would remain in the repertoire long after other specific clones had senesced. TCC die by apoptosis in vitro at the end of their lifespans, and if this also occurs in vivo they would thus be subject to peripheral clonal deletion from the repertoire. There is evidence from studies of human T cells ex vivo in the elderly that both repertoire restriction and increased clonal deletion by apoptosis do indeed occur.

Table 1 **T cell longevity in culture**

Origin	CE%	n, clones/expts	Percentage of clones reaching population size: 20 PD (10^6)	30 PD (10^9)	40 PD (10^{12})	longest-lived
CD34+	59	581 / 7	32	18	7%	60 PD
CD34+ (cord)	43	94 / 2	29	nyat		57
CD3+ (y, HS)	45	1372 / 15	42	21	15	170
CD3+ (old, HS)	0	0 / 6	0			
CD3+ (y, X-V)	86	96 / 1	32	nyat		48
CD3+ (old, X-V)	52	116 / 2	55	nyat		41

CE, cloning efficiency (calculated from percentage of wells positive in cloning plates). Longevity is expressed as a percentage of established clones (ie. those counted as positive in calculating the CE) which survive to 20, 30 or 40 PD. $CD34^+$, positively selected stem cells; $CD3^-CD7^+$, T cell progenitors; $CD3^+$, normal peripheral T cells; y(oung) and old, apparently healthy donors under 30 yr. and SENIEUR-selected donors over 95 yr., respectively; HS, human serum; X-V, X-Vivo 10 medium. nyat = not yet all tested.

3. Cloning of T cells from the very elderly

Accumulated evidence suggests that T cell function in the elderly is compromised, and that certain biomarkers of ageing may be associated with this (eg. decreased expression of CD28, decreased telomere lengths, decreased secretion of IL 2). However, in strictly selected perfectly healthy elderly donors, many but not all of the age-associated T cell alterations observed in the general elderly population are no longer present. We were therefore interested to investigate whether the characteristics of TCC derived from these healthy elderly donors were different from those previously established using young donors (eg. because elderly donors′ T cells may have proliferated extensively already in vivo before cloning). First experiments supported this possibility, because cloning T cells from old (>95 yr) SENIEUR donors using the same culture conditions as used successfully for young donors′ T cells (RPMI 1640 + 10% human serum and IL 2) failed to result in the generation of any clones at all (Table 1), although their responses in mixed lymphocyte cultures (MLC) had not been found to be markedly decreased in a small series of experiments (data not shown). This finding was consistent with the hypothesis that T cell ageing may have occurred in vivo such that the replicative lifespan of the clones in vivo was already close to exhaustion. However, we now know that this cannot be the case, because cloning and culture in a recently developed serum-free medium (X-Vivo 10, BioWhittaker) has enabled equally high cloning efficiencies to be obtained even in near-centenarians as in the young. This is the first time that it has been possible to clone and culture T cells in serum-free medium, after many attempts in the past [9]. As far as these serum-free culture experiments have been taken, it is possible to say that the proportion of clones achieving 20 PD is in fact very similar in the old and young donors. Moreover, the maximum lifespans of that fraction of clones which has already been cultured up to the end of their lifespans to date also seem very comparable. Although all the data on average clonal longevities are not yet in, this therefore suggests that even very old perfectly healthy donors possess T cells with an intact replicative capacity compared to young donors. This may imply 1) that senescent cells have not been accumulating in these (albeit rare, highly selected nonagenarian SENIEUR) donors and 2) that, unlike T cells from young donors, the growth of T cells from old donors is not supported by pooled human serum (here derived predominantly from young or middle-aged males).

4. Extrathymic T cell differentiation

It seems, therefore, that at the extreme of exceptionally healthy old age (but not necessarily averagely healthy old-age), T cells in this system behave comparably whether derived from old or young donors (at least regarding their culture longevity). It was therefore of interest to investigate whether T cells of extreme youth behaved any differently. In this case, the hypothesis was that they would manifest increased longevities as a result of not having divided previously in vivo. For these experiments we used CD34+ cells from cord blood of new-borns or normal young healthy adults. We had first established extra-thymic T cell differentation systems using T cells progenitors [10,11], and, most recently, extended this system to $CD34^+$ stem cells [12]. The results of these experiments so far are also summarized in Table 1, which shows longevities of TCC derived from these two types of extrathymic T cell differentiation system. In contrast to our hypothesis (and earlier data which had suggested that T cells from the first of these sources did experience longer average lifespans in vitro), it seems from these more extensive data that the life expectancies of such T cells are if anything lower than those of TCC derived from mature T cells. This seems to imply that (these variable) lifespans are determined by culture conditions rather than origins. However, the process is not entirely stochastic because short-lived and long-lived TCC cryopreserved at an early passage retain their characteristic longevity profile when thawed and cultured further (Pawelec, unpublished results). A burning question, therefore, is what "programs" these markedly different longevities in culture, if not the previous proliferative history of the cell? One possibility is that the previous proliferative history of the *stem* cell does so. There is indeed a body of data consistent with this possibility, discussed in detail in our on-line review at www.bioscience.org (Frontiers of Bioscience 4, d216, 1999). Others might argue that this type of culture-determined longevity supports the idea that ageing in vitro is an artefact not relevant to in vivo phenomena [6]. We were therefore anxious to monitor structural and functional alterations to these T cells during culture (rather than simply measuring the time at which they stopped growing and died) because if characteristics of ageing in vitro could be validated in vivo, it would be unlikely that the "ageing" process in vitro was a culture artefact. The identification of causative factors, moreover, which might allow manipulations of conditions to extend longevity in vitro might provide a rational for attempts to prevent or reverse immunosenescence in vivo.

5. Biomarkers of ageing: surface marker phenotyping

Monoclonal antibodies are now available in great abundance to a wide range of surface molecules on T cells, and flow cytometry offers a convenient technique for surveying large numbers of molecules the quantitative expression of which may change with age. However, this approach is more complicated perhaps than generally appreciated. Distinguishing between changes associated with growth and activation status of cells and their age is a major challenge. For comparison of data sets, there are also two possible ways of considering the age of the cells: either as the absolute number of PD undergone or in terms of the fraction of each clone's lifespan completed. Our most extensive analysis so far has been confined to the former, ie. by comparing "young" cells and "old" cells from the same clones. However, it should be pointed out that the "young" cells in these experiments were still older than the average lifespan even of established clones. Clearly, we are only dealing with a subset of clones which anyway tend to have greater than average longevity. In this context, it seems that the expression of most surface markers does not change with culture age. Thus, the density of expression of many of the surface structures known to be critical for the activation of T cells did not change markedly or consistently. This statement applies to the specific antigen receptor itself, a whole range of accessory/adhesion molecules such as CD54, CD58 etc., as well as CD45R family molecules and for most clones, CD95 as well. Given the heterogeneity of the clones, however, these findings do not exclude that age-associated alterations in the expression of these molecules might be observed on certain individual clones, and we have indeed observed this. For example, certain rare clones with a low level of CD95 show increased levels of CD95 with ageing. Thus far it has not proven possible to assign any particular significance to such changes or to identify any characteristics differences between TCC which show such changes and those which do not. However, some age-associated changes have indeed been observed in the majority of (but never all) clones in the expression of certain cell surface structures. One common finding was a reduction in the density of expression of CD28, CD134 and CD154 [13]. Interestingly, all three of these molecules have been implicated in accessory signalling to the T cell ("costimulation"). In addition, expression of CD154 (CD40-ligand) may be required to fully activate antigen-presenting cells to become sufficiently potent stimulators to activate the TCC. This possibility is supported by the finding that "senescent" T cells can still be restimulated by fully activated dendritic cells even after they have lost the ability to respond to "conventional" stimulators [14]. In the case of CD28, prior to senescence, its level of expression commonly fell so low as to be undetectable by FACS, and a functional consequence of this was that the degree of autocrine proliferation of the cells decreased as the level of CD28 decreased [8]. We also observed decreased expression of IL 2, IL 4 and IL 7 receptors on the majority of clones, possibly secondary to decreased costimulation [13]. Moreover, not only were decreases in the level of expression of certain cell surface molecules recorded, but also increases in expression of others. Thus, the density of expression of the negative costimulatory receptor CD152 (CTLA-4) and of the "killer-inhibitory receptor" CD94 was increased on some of the clones as they aged (Pawelec et al., unpublished results). We therefore searched the literature for evidence that similar changes occurred in vivo in an age-associated manner. For CD28 expression there is increasing evidence that this is indeed the case, both on CD4 and CD8 cells. Moreover, in many different pathological conditions sharing only the characteristics of chronic antigenic stimulation in vivo, the number of cells expressing CD28 is reported to be decreased (reviewed in [15]). Regarding CD94 and CD134, no reports on age-associated change in vivo seem to have appeared thus far. However, age-associated decreased expression CD154 on human T cells was recently reported in two separate publications [16,17], and in mouse there is one report of increased CD152 expression [18].

6. Functional consequences: Cytokine secretion

T cell ageing in our in vitro system is characterised by a progressive loss of ability to undergo autocrine proliferation some time before replicative senescence occurs. At this time, TCC can still be maintained with exogenous IL 2 but no longer secrete it in large amounts. Nonetheless, old cells from TCC retain antigen-specific TCR function, as shown by their retention of ability to secrete cytokines such as IFN-γ, and enhanced ability to secrete IL 10 [13]. Decreased IL 2 secretion coupled with increased IL 10 (as well as possibly increased TGF-ß, unpublished results) and more or less constant IFN-γ production quite accurately reflects a consensus of studies published over the years on cytokine secretion from freshly isolated cells in the elderly (reviewed in [15]).

7. Functional consequences: Apoptosis induction

Old CD4+ TCC manifest an age-associated (rather slight) increase of susceptibility to activation-induced cell death (AICD) prior to their eventual final clonal deletion by apoptosis [19]. This may also be related to decreased levels of CD28 expression and decreased IL 2 secretion. However, even in the presence of exogenous IL 2, they show increased susceptibility to AICD, which is mediated by fas/fas-ligand interactions. The clones do not generally show an age-associated increase in the density of CD95 expression as mentioned above; however, they may more consistently show an age-related increase in fas-ligand mRNA which could contribute to enhanced susceptibility to AICD (M. Adibzadeh, unpublished results). The situation in vivo is not yet completely clear from the literature. While all studies published report increased susceptibility to apoptosis of CD4+ cells; there is disagreement on CD8 with some claiming increased, others decreased, apoptosis. There is clearly a tendency towards increased apoptosis with age [20-24]. These results are more fully discussed in our on-line review at www.bioscience.org (Frontiers of Bioscience 4, d216, 1999).

8. Cytotoxicity

Under standard culture conditions, it is difficult or impossible to detect cytotoxic activity of these alloreactive Th0-like TCC. However, as they age in culture, lytic activity towards NK-susceptible target cells may develop [25]. This is greatly facilitated by exposure of the cells to high concentrations of IL 2; indeed, NK-like cytotoxicity can be induced even in young clones by a relatively short period of culture with IL 2 [26]. Culture with large amounts of IL 4, on the other hand, while also able to enhance cytotoxic activity, did not result in NK-like activity but rather increased allospecific activity [26]. These results are interpreted to mean that Th0 cells possess the potential for cytotoxic activity which can be visualized by altering the cytokine environment (and can also be developed in young clones using lectin). Acquisition of measurable cytotoxicity with age may then represent the result of cumulative exposure to low levels of cytokines that mimics the effects of shorter exposure to larger amounts of cytokine. This is a good example of what we originally termed the "functional flexibility" of T cells [27].

9. Negative regulation

The majority of young CD4 TCR2+ Th0-like TCC possess helper function for B cell Ig synthesis and do not inhibit the proliferative responses of other TCC when admixed with them or when their supernatants are added to such cultures [28]. However, ageing of the TCC in vitro results in downregulation of B cell helper activity and may even result in the acquisition of an active suppressive effect in mixed cultures [25]. It was suggested that such suppressive activity was an artefact created by mycoplasma contamination of the cell cultures [29], but there are several reasons for rejecting this explanation: 1) anti-mycoplasma agents fail to prevent it and there is no evidence for mycoplasma contamination of the cultures [25], 2) subcloning of the TCC prior to or after acquisition of suppressive activity results in the isolation of some subclones with and some without suppressive activity [30], 3) subsubcloning non-suppressive subclones reproduces this effect (unpublished), 4) in systems for measuring suppression where cell/cell contact is required, certain MHC class II-specific mAb could block inhibitory activities [31].

The inhibitory activity for Ig production or for autocrine proliferative responses is contained in the supernatants from old clones and may be partly attributed to cytokines such as IL 10, which is produced in greater abundance as TCC age. IL 10 is a pleiotropic cytokine secreted by Th1 and Th2 cells in man [32] as well as by Th0 cells and inhibits immune responses by several different mechanisms [33]. However, it also has positive effects on T cell responses, particularly because of its anti-apoptotic effects [34] which can even result in sufficient continued short-term proliferation of T cells for this to be registered as thymidine incorporation [35]. When considering its role in immunosenescence it is important to note that in young TCC, culture with IL 10 can result in anergy induction [36]. Anergy is a state to some extent resembling senescence in terms of its hallmark blockade of IL 2 gene transcription, although different in terms of IL 2-responsiveness [37]. Increased levels of IL 10 production by old TCC might therefore contribute to downregulation of the T cell response both by its effects on the producer cells as well as bystander effects on other cells (ie. suppression). It is also worth remembering that several reports have indicated that young TCC purposefully rendered anergic do exert suppressive effects on other, non-anergic, cells [38].

However, at least one other mechanism for suppression is active in these cells; this requires cell/cell contact. As TCC age in culture they retain similar densities of expression of MHC class II HLA-DR, DQ and DP molecules as young cells, yet reactivity with certain broadly reactive anti-class II mAb such as SG520 and TÜ39 increases [39]. This "extra" reactivity, which can be precipitated from sequentially DR, DQ and DP-precleared cell lysates [31] appears identical to HLA-DR on 2-D gels [40]. Despite attempts to characterize this moiety by protein sequencing and molecular genetic means, its exact identity has remained elusive. Others who have reported possibly similar types of data have also thus far not been able to clarify exactly what this is [41,42]. Protein sequencing data have suggested that there is no relationship between this moiety, termed "DY" and either HLA-DM or invariant chain (H. Pohla et al., unpublished results). We are currently pursuing the hypothesis that it might represent a particular association of HLA-DR molecules at the surface [43], as a dimer of heterdimers, or "superdimer" (Fernandez & Pawelec, unpublished). Whatever the exact nature of this entity, it is proposed that it participates in the generation of autoreactive negative regulatory variants within or between monoclonal populations. The data on which this idea is based are as follows: old TCC express larger amounts of this entity than young TCC [39]; old TCC but not young cells from the same clones can induce suppressive activity in autologous PBMC [25]; this induction event can be blocked by broadly reactive class II-specific mAb such as SG520 and Tü39, but not by monospecific HLA-DR, DQ or DP mAb [31]. It is therefore proposed that the increased levels of expression of this putative class II molecule on the surface of aged T cells may contribute to their own as well as bystander T cell downregulation [44].

10. Is telomerase expression a biomarker of ageing in human TCC?

Telomere attrition as a possible causative mechanism of replicative senescence in fibroblasts has been intensively investigated over the past few years. However, relatively little is known of telomere length dynamics in T cells and even less on telomerase regulation. It is clear that, unlike fibroblasts, stimulated T cells can upregulate telomerase and possibly maintain telomere lengths for at least a limited period during which they proliferate. Telomerase activity is regulated in the G1 phase of the cell cycle in normal human T cells, as indicated by the finding that rapamycin (which blocks TCR-signal transduction and cdk2 activation) but not hydroxyurea (an S-phase inhibitor) prevents telomerase induction [45]. Telomerase is upregulated by T cells within 24 h., increases up to 72 h. and then decreases again after 96 h if the cells are not restimulated [46]. Telomere lengths do not decrease during this period, but possibly because telomerase is downregulated again, decreases in telomere length are not prevented during long-term culture, although they may be prevented initially [47]. In CD8 cells, Monteiro et al. [48] reported that telomere lengths in the CD28-negative population were shorter than in the CD28+ CD8+ population, and that in vitro clonal expansion of CD8 cells is associated with telomere shortening. Optimal telomerase induction requires optimal stimulation via CD3 and CD28 [49], so age-associated defects in CD28 may also contribute to suboptimal telomerase induction. Pan et al. reported that telomerase was upregulated in normal PBMC after their stimulation with PHA [50]. Continued culture of these cells with IL 2 resulted in eventual cessation of growth after ca. 23 PD, when telomerase activity was no longer found. Confusingly, the authors interpreted this as demonstrating downregulation of telomerase at senescence. However, they presented no evidence that their T cells were in fact senescent; they had ceased proliferation because they were not restimulated via the TCR. Thus, they merely demonstrated that telomerase expression correlates with proliferation of the T cells. Consistent with this interpretation, they also mentioned a T cell clone which they did maintain by intermittent restimulation, and here they showed the presence of telomerase in stimulated cells and its absence in "resting" cells [50]. Thus, the increase in telomerase activity after stimulation is transient but may be upregulated in certain clones at least upon restimulation. In uncloned CD4 cells intermittently stimulated with CD3 and CD28 mAb, the initial strong telomerase upregulation was found to be weaker at each restimulation until it was no longer upregulated at all; at this point, telomere lengths of the cultured cells decreased [51]. Similarly, in CD8+ cells, it has been found that the degree to which telomerase activity is upregulated after repeated stimulation of antigen-specific T cells was inversely related to the length of time that they had been in culture (Valenzuela & Effros, manuscript in preparation). Whether the situation is comparable in vivo is open to question. In acute infectious mononucleosis it was found that CD8 cells upregulate telomerase and maintain or even increase telomere lengths until resolution of infection [3]. Thus, the conditions for up and downregulation of telomerase and the maintenance of an effective level of telomerase in T cells are not clearly defined so far, but may be critical to the fate of the responding T cells and thence to the T cell-mediated immune response itself. In certain cases of apparent immortalization of abnormal (but non-tumorigenic) human T cells, telomerase was found not to be downregulated; its high level of expression, as found in the majority of tumors, may be responsible for the extended longevity of these T cells [52]. In some way, these cultures perhaps parallel the in vivo situation in AIM more closely.

Telomerase may not be the only factor determining telomere length and cell survival. Strahl & Blackburn reported [53] that inhibitors of retroviral reverse transcriptase (telomerase itself is a specialized cellular reverse transcriptase) could cause progressive telomere shortening of immortalized human lymphoid cell lines in vitro. Telomerase activity was present in these lines and its activity was blocked by the agents tested. Telomeres in the blocked lines eventually stabilized and remained short. It was, however, suggested that telomere lengths in lymphoid cells lines (which were unstable even in the absence of inhibitors) are determined both by telomerase and telomerase-independent mechanisms. More recent data have confirmed and taken this idea further [54]. On the other hand, certain tissues appear to undergo senescence correlated to decreased telomerase activity despite their ability to maintain telomere lengths [55]. However, that both telomerase activity and telomere length can be absolutely critical in determining longevity of cells in culture has been unequivocally demonstrated by two independent laboratories [56,57] and indirectly confirmed by a third [58]. Using telomerase-negative cell types, they found that transfection of the gene for the catalytic component of telomerase extended life-span way beyond the point at which untransfected lines senesced. This life-span extension was not accompanied by acquisition of abnormal karyotype or surface markers, but was associated with telomere length extension and inhibited expression of the senescence-associated ß-galactosidase marker. This is the first evidence for a causal relationship between telomere shortening and cellular senescence in vitro.

In the TCC studied here, we have shown that telomerase reinduction occurs in parallel with autocrine proliferation. Stimulation results in the rapid upregulation of telomerase in young cells, and this is further enhanced, and the kinetic extended, in the presence of exogenous IL 2 (Fig. 1). However, later passage cells from the same clone no longer upregulate telomerase even in the presence of IL 2 (Fig. 1). It is at this time point that stimulation no longer results in proliferation (Fig. 2), and telomerase activity can no longer be detected (Fig. 1). Moreover, as illustrated in the Figs., the parallel loss of both autocrine proliferative capacity and telomerase induction also occurs in clones which senesce at an early passage number, as well as those senescing at later passages (data not shown). These findings may suggest that telomerase is a marker for T cell activation rather than being instrumental in preventing triggering growth arrest of the cells, but this hypothesis still requires testing. Further studies are required to clarify the role of telomerase and its mechanism of induction, and whether telomere attrition in lymphocytes is really an effector mechanism of cellular senescence. Nonetheless, in vivo, an age-associated reduction in telomere lengths is observed [59] and telomere attrition occurs more rapidly in premature aging syndromes [60,61]. Weng et al. [62] reported that $CD4^+$ memory-phenotype cells showed consistently shorter telomeres than naive-phenotype cells. Interestingly, this difference in telomere length between naive- and memory-phenotype cells was the same whether the cells were isolated from young or old donors. These data do suggest a role for telomere attrition in T cell ageing and once again indicate that the in vitro and in vivo data are more closely in agreement than disagreement.

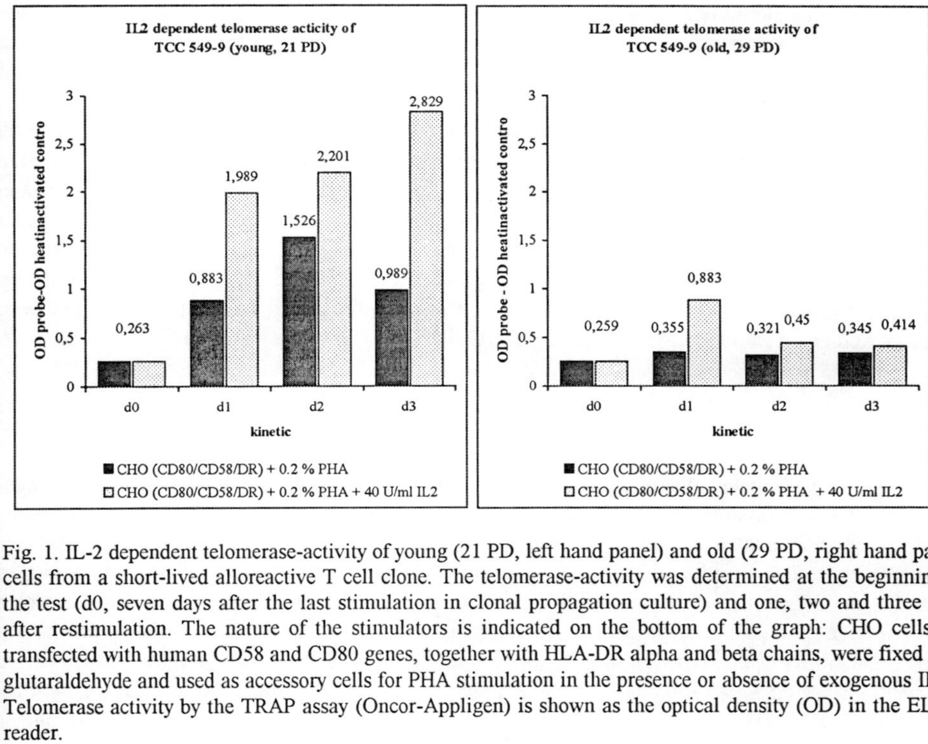

Fig. 1. IL-2 dependent telomerase-activity of young (21 PD, left hand panel) and old (29 PD, right hand panel) cells from a short-lived alloreactive T cell clone. The telomerase-activity was determined at the beginning of the test (d0, seven days after the last stimulation in clonal propagation culture) and one, two and three days after restimulation. The nature of the stimulators is indicated on the bottom of the graph: CHO cells co-transfected with human CD58 and CD80 genes, together with HLA-DR alpha and beta chains, were fixed with glutaraldehyde and used as accessory cells for PHA stimulation in the presence or absence of exogenous IL 2. Telomerase activity by the TRAP assay (Oncor-Appligen) is shown as the optical density (OD) in the ELISA reader.

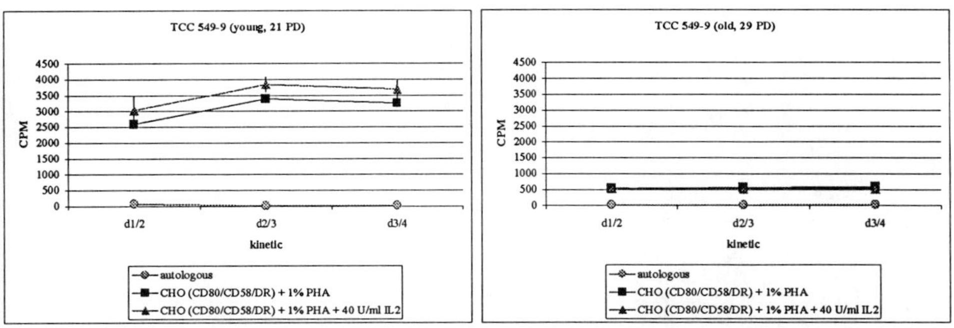

Figure 2: Proliferation-kinetic of young (21 PD, left hand panel) and senescent (29 PD, right hand panel) cells from the same short-lived clone as in Fig. 1. The proliferation was measured by [^{3}H]-thymidine incorporation after 42 h, 66 h or 90 h (day 1/2, 2/3 and 3/4 respectively) using the same stimulators as in Fig. 1.

11. Expression of mitotic inhibitors

Telomere attrition may trigger growth arrest by activating DNA damage limitation programs. Growth arrest mediated by mitotic inhibitors allows time for DNA repair mechanisms to attempt to make good the damage (see Barnett et al., this volume). In the case of telomere attrition they obviously cannnot repair this type of "damage" and so apoptosis is triggered to delete the potentially dangerous, neoplastic, cell. Preliminary results of experiments carried out as part of the EUCAMBIS collaborative workshop examined the expression of mRNA for p16-^{INK4a}, p21^{sdi} and p27^{kip} in cells from young and old TCC (see Chapter 1). Cells from old TCC were found to contain more message for all three mitotic inhibitors than young cells. In the case of p21, no message at all was detectable in the young cells. Although it was previously thought that p16 was not expressed in T cells, more recent work by Erickson et al. showed that both p16 and p15 proteins accumulate, whereas p21 levels were only slightly elevated, as PHA-stimulated T cells age in culture, and that there was increased binding of p16 to its target Cdk6 kinase [63]. Therefore, p16 may play an important role in growth control of lymphocytes as well and could be a target for manipulation in immunosenescence. The situation ex vivo in T cells from the young and old has not yet been properly studied. Preliminary data from the EUCAMBIS study are given in Chapter 1.

12. Conclusions

The in vitro behaviour of cultured T cells at the clonal level is an accurate model for age-associated T cell alterations in vivo (Table 2). It may be possible to employ clonal T cell cultures to search for age-associated characteristics representing risk factors for immunosenescence in vivo. Furthermore, screening approaches to manipulate immunosenescence in vivo may be developed using this in vitro model. At the simplest level, this could be testing the effects of hormones, vitamin and mineral supplements, anti-oxidants etc. An understanding of and ability to influence the up- and down-regulation of CD28 and CD152, as well as CD134 and CD154 might also result in interventions to enhance immunity in the elderly. In addition, attempts to increase functional longevity of the T cells by more invasive manipulations such as enforcing expression of telomerase or blockade of mitotic inhibitors at the same time as enhancing DNA repair capacity might be an option [64].

Table 2 **Possible similarities between in vivo and in vitro T cell ageing**

Decreased	Increased
↓ CD28 expression	↑ p27
↓ CD154 expression	↑ p16
↓ IL 2R expression	↑ mutation frequency
↓ IL 2 production	↑ CD152 expression
↓ bcl-2	↑ IL 10 production
↓ telomere lengths	↑ DNA damage
↓ telomerase induction	↑ apoptosis
↓ CD134	
↓ DNA repair	
↓ stress resistance and HSP expression	
↓ TCR signalling	

13. Acknowledgements

Support for the work from the author's laboratory, and the EUCAMBIS project, discussed here came from the Deutsche Forschungsgemeinschaft, the VERUM Foundation, the Mildred Scheel Foundation, the Sandoz Foundation for Gerontological Research, and the European Commission (BMHI-CT94-1209; project EUCAMBIS; BMH4-CT98-3058; project EUCAPS).

14. References

[1] G. Pawelec, R. Solana, E. Remarque, et al., Impact of aging on innate immunity. J. Leukocyte Biol. J Leuk Biol 64 (1998) 703-712.

[2] M.M. Steger, C. Maczek and B. Grubeck-Loebenstein, Morphologically and functionally intact dendritic cells can be derived from the peripheral blood of aged individuals. Clin. Exp. Immunol. 105 (1996) 544-550.

[3] M.K. Maini, M.V.D. Soares, C.F. Zilch, et al., Virus-induced CD8+ T cell clonal expansion is associated with telomerase up-regulation and telomere length preservation: A mechanism for rescue from replicative senescence. J. Immunol. 162 (1999) 4521-4526.

[4] L. Bruno, J. Kirberg and H. Von Boehmer, On the cellular basis of immunological T cell memory. Immunity 2 (1995) 37-43.

[5] R.B. Effros and G. Pawelec, Replicative senescence of T lymphocytes: does the Hayflick Limit lead to immune exhaustion? Immunol. Today 18 (1997) 450-454.

[6] H. Rubin, Telomere-dependent senescence - Reply. Nat. Biotechnol. 17 (1999) 313-314.

[7] M. McCarron, Y. Osborne, C. Story, et al., Effect of age on lymphocyte proliferation. Mech. Ageing Dev. 41 (1987) 211-218.

[8] M. Adibzadeh, H. Pohla, A. Rehbein, et al., Long-term culture of monoclonal human T lymphocytes: models for immunosenescence? Mech. Ageing Dev. 83 (1995) 171-183.

[9] G. Pawelec (1993): Cloning and propagation of human T lymphocytes. In: Tumour Immunobiology. A Practical Approach. (Eds: G. Gallagher, R.C. Rees and C.W. Reynolds) IRL Press, Oxford, 131-141.

[10] H. Pohla, M. Adibzadeh, H.J. Buhring, et al., Evolution of a CD3+CD4+ alpha/beta T-Cell Receptor Plus Mature T-Cell Clone from CD3-CD7+ Sorted Human Bone Marrow Cells. Dev. Immunol. 3 (1993) 197-210.

[11] M. Adibzadeh, H.J. Buhring, T. Daikeler, et al., Extrathymic Development and Function of Human T-Lymphocytes from Bone Marrow Cells in Vitro. Cell. Immunol. 154 (1994) 25-42.

[12] G. Pawelec, R. Müller, A. Rehbein, et al., Extrathymic T cell differentiation in vitro from CD34+ stem cells. J. Leukocyte Biol. 64 (1998) 733-739.

[13] G. Pawelec, A. Rehbein, K. Haehnel, et al., Human T cell clones as a model for immunosenescence. Immunol. Rev. 160 (1997) 31-43.

[14] M.M. Steger, C. Maczek and B. Grubeck-Loebenstein, Peripheral blood dendritic cells reinduce proliferation in in vitro aged T cell populations. Mech. Ageing Dev. 93 (1997) 125-130.

[15] G. Pawelec, W. Wagner, M. Adibzadeh, et al., T cell immunosenescence in vitro and in vivo. Exp. Gerontol. 34 (1999) 419-429.

[16] C.M. Weyand, J.C. Brandes, D. Schmidt, et al., Functional properties of CD4+CD28- T cells in the aging immune system. Mech. Ageing Dev. 102 (1998) 131-147.

[17] D. Lio, C. D'Anna, F. Gervasi, et al., Interleukin 12-release by mitogen-stimulated mononuclear cells in the elderly. Mech. Ageing Dev. 102 (1998) 211-219.

[18] A. Wakikawa, M. Utsuyama and K. Hirokawa, Altered expression of various receptors on T cells in young and old mice after mitogenic stimulation: A flow cytometric analysis. Mech. Ageing Dev. 94 (1997) 113-122.

[19] G. Pawelec, D. Sansom, A. Rehbein, et al., Decreased proliferative capacity and increased susceptibility to activation-induced cell death in late-passage human CD4+ TCR2+ cultured T cell clones. Exp. Gerontol. 31 (1996) 655-668.

[20] T. Miyawaki, T. Uehara, R. Nibu, et al., Differential Expression of Apoptosis-Related Fas Antigen on Lymphocyte Subpopulations in Human Peripheral Blood. J. Immunol. 149 (1992) 3753-3758.

[21] S. Shinohara, T. Sawada, Y. Nishioka, et al., Differential expression of Fas antigen and bcl-2 protein on CD4+ T cells, CD8+ T cells, and monocytes. Cell. Immunol. 163 (1995) 303-308.

[22] M.A. Phelouzat, T. Laforge, A. Arbogast, et al., Susceptibility to apoptosis of T lymphocytes from elderly humans is associated with increased in vivo expression of functional Fas receptors. Mech. Ageing Dev. 96 (1997) 35-46.

[23] R. Aspinall, J. Carroll and S.S. Jiang, Age-related changes in the absolute number of CD95 positive cells in T cell subsets in the blood. Exp. Gerontol. 33 (1998) 581-591.

[24] S. Aggarwal and S. Gupta, Increased apoptosis of T cell subsets in aging humans: Altered expression of Fas (CD95), Fas ligand, Bcl-2, and Bax. J. Immunol. 160 (1998) 1627-1637.

[25] G. Pawelec, E.M. Schneider and P. Wernet, Acquisition of suppressive activity and natural killer-like cytotoxicity by human alloproliferative "helper" T cell clones. J. Immunol. 136 (1986) 402-411.

[26] G. Pawelec, Modulation of IL-2- and IL-4-induced cytotoxicities in human T helper lymphocyte clones by tumor necrosis factor-α. J. Immunol. 146 (1991) 572-576.

[27] G. Pawelec, E.M. Schneider and P. Wernet, Human T-cell clones with multiple and changing functions: indications of unexpected flexibility in immune respons networks. Immunology Today. 4 (1983) 275-278.

[28] F. Falcioni, G. Pawelec, N. Brattig, et al., Functionally distinct human T-lymphocyte clones sharing potent suppressive activity on immunoglobulin secretion. Immunology 54 (1985) 685-692.

[29] S. Rosen-Bronson and D.D. Eckels, Longevity of human allospecific TLCs: mycoplasma infection as the cause of in vitro "suppression" of MLC. Human Immunol. 14 (1985) 365-377.

[30] P. Wernet, E.M. Schneider, F. Kalthoff, et al., Constitutive functional heterogeneity without detectable somatic mutation of antigen receptor genes in helper T cell clones: possible regulation by novel HLA class II "DY" determinants. Immunol. Rev. 96 (1987) 109-140.

[31] G. Pawelec, N. Fernandez, T. Brocker, et al., DY determinants, possibly associated with novel class II molecules, stimulate autoreactive CD4+ T cells with suppressive activity. J. Exp. Med. 167 (1988) 243-261.

[32] G. Del Prete, M. Decarli, F. Almerigogna, et al., Human IL-10 Is Produced by Both Type-1 Helper (Th1) and Type-2 Helper (Th2) T-Cell Clones and Inhibits Their Antigen-Specific Proliferation and Cytokine Production. J. Immunol. 150 (1993) 353-360.

[33] K.W. Moore, A. O'Garra, R.D. Malefyt, et al., Interleukin-10. Annu. Rev. Immunol. 11 (1993) 165-190.

[34] K. Taga, B. Cherney and G. Tosato, IL-10 Inhibits Apoptotic Cell Death in Human T-Cells Starved of IL-2. Int. Immunol. 5 (1993) 1599-1608.

[35] G. Pawelec, H. Pohla, E. Schlotz, et al., Interleukin 10 is a human T cell growth factor in vitro. Cytokine 7 (1995) 355-363.

[36] J.C. Becker, C. Czerny and E.B. Brocker, Maintenance of clonal anergy by endogenously produced IL-10. Int. Immunol. 6 (1994) 1605-1612.

[37] J.R. Lamb, B.J. Skidmore, N. Green, et al., Induction of tolerance in influenza virus-immune T lymphocyte clones with synthetic peptides of influenza hemagglutinin. J. Exp. Med. 157 (1983) 1434-1447.

[38] G. Lombardi, S. Sidhu, R. Batchelor, et al., Anergic T cells as suppressor cells in vitro. Science 264 (1994) 1587-1589.

[39] N. Fernandez, M. Kurpisz, M. Labeta, et al., A Ligand-Epitope Invitro Analysis of Major Histocompatibility Determinants Expressed on Lymphocyte-B and Lymphocyte-T. Immunol. 77 (1992) 116-122.

[40] N. Fernandez, M.O. Labeta and H. Festenstein, A novel HLA class II molecule. Immunogenetics 27 (1988) 363-369.

[41] D. Santoli, S.F. Radka, M. Igarashi, et al., Autlogous B-lymphoblastoid cell lines and long-term cultured T cells as stimulators in the mixed lymphocyte reaction: analysis of the role of HLA class II antigens as stimulatory molecules. J. Immunol. 137 (1986) 400-407.

[42] G. Carra, M. Giunta, C. Benati, et al., Selective association of a 22-38 kDa glycoprotein with MHC class II DP antigen on activated human lymphocytes at the plasma membrane. Mol. Immunol. 33 (1996) 269-278.

[43] K.M. Wilson, I.E.G. Morrison, P.R. Smith, et al., Single particle tracking of cell-surface HLA-DR molecules using R-phycoerythrin labeled monoclonal antibodies and fluorescence digital imaging. J. Cell Sci. 109 (1996) 2101-2109.

[44] G. Pawelec, T. Brocker, F.W. Busch, et al., "Tolerisation" of human T-helper cell clones by chronic exposure to alloantigen: culture conditions dictate autocrine proliferative status but not acquisition of cytotoxic potential and suppressor-induction capacity. J. Mol. Cell. Immunol. 4 (1988) 21-34.

[45] K.J. Buchkovich and C.W. Greider, Telomerase regulation during entry into the cell cycle in normal human T cells. Mol. Biol. Cell 7 (1996) 1443-1454.

[46] O. Yamada, T. Motoji and H. Mizoguchi, Up-regulation of telomerase activity in human lymphocytes. Bba-Mol. Cell. Res. 1314 (1996) 260-266.

[47] A.G. Bodnar, N.W. Kim, R.B. Effros, et al., Mechanism of telomerase induction during T cell activation. Exp. Cell Res. 228 (1996) 58-64.

[48] J. Monteiro, F. Batliwalla, H. Ostrer, et al., Shortened telomeres in clonally expanded CD28-CD8+ T cells imply a replicative history that is distinct from their CD28+CD8+ counterparts. J. Immunol. 156 (1996) 3587-3590.

[49] K.S. Hathcock, N.P. Weng, R. Merica, et al., Antigen-dependent regulation of telomerase activity in murine T cells. J. Immunol. 160 (1998) 5702-5706.

[50] C.G. Pan, B.H. Xue, T.M. Ellis, et al., Changes in telomerase activity and telomere length during human T lymphocyte senescence. Exp. Cell Res. 231 (1997) 346-353.

[51] N.P. Weng, L.D. Palmer, B.L. Levine, et al., Tales of tails: Regulation of telomere length and telomerase activity during lymphocyte development, differentiation, activation, and aging. Immunol. Rev. 160 (1997) 43-54.

[52] K. Kaltoft, Cytokine-driven immortalization of in vitro activated human T lymphocytes - CD28 expression correlates inversely with cell population doublings. Exp. Clin. Immunogenet. 15 (1998) 84-89.

[53] C. Strahl and E.H. Blackburn, Effects of reverse transcriptase inhibitors on telomere length and telomerase activity in two immortalized human cell lines. Mol. Cell. Biol. 16 (1996) 53-65.

[54] T.M. Bryan, A. Englezou, L. Dallapozza, et al., Evidence for an alternative mechanism for maintaining telomere length in human tumors and tumor-derived cell lines. Nature Med. 3 (1997) 1271-1274.

[55] M.K. Kang, W.T. Guo and N.H. Park, Replicative senescence of normal human oral keratinocytes is associated with the loss of telomerase activity without shortening of telomeres. Cell Growth Differ. 9 (1998) 85-95.

[56] H. Vaziri and S. Benchimol, Reconstitution of telomerase activity in normal human cells leads to elongation of telomeres and extended replicative life span. Curr. Biol. 8 (1998) 279-282.

[57] A.G. Bodnar, M. Ouellette, M. Frolkis, et al., Extension of life-span by introduction of telomerase into normal human cells. Science 279 (1998) 349-352.

[58] C.M. Counter, M. Meyerson, E.N. Eaton, et al., Telomerase activity is restored in human cells by ectopic expression of hTERT (hEST2), the catalytic subunit of telomerase. Oncogene 16 (1998) 1217-1222.

[59] P.E. Slagboom, S. Droog and D.I. Boomsma, Genetic determination of telomere size in humans: A twin study of three age groups. Am. J. Hum. Genet. 55 (1994) 876-882.

[60] R.C. Allsopp, H. Vaziri, C. Patterson, et al., Telomere Length Predicts Replicative Capacity of Human Fibroblasts. Proc. Natl. Acad. Sci. USA 89 (1992) 10114-10118.

[61] H. Vaziri, F. Schachter, I. Uchida, et al., Loss of Telomeric DNA During Aging of Normal and Trisomy-21 Human Lymphocytes. Am. J. Hum. Genet. 52 (1993) 661-667.

[62] N.P. Weng, B.L. Levine, C.H. June, et al., Human naive and memory T lymphocytes differ in telomeric length and replicative potential. Proc. Natl. Acad. Sci. USA 92 (1995) 11091-11094.

[63] S. Erickson, O. Sangfelt, M. Heyman, et al., Involvement of the Ink4 proteins p16 and p15 in T-lymphocyte senescence. Oncogene 17 (1998) 595-602.

[64] T. Moritz, W. Mackay, B.J. Glassner, et al., Retrovirus-mediated expression of a DNA repair protein in bone marrow protects hematopoietic cells from nitrosourea-induced toxicity in vitro and in vivo. Cancer Res. 55 (1995) 2608-2614.

EUCAMBIS: Immunology and Ageing in Europe
G. Pawelec (Ed.)
IOS Press, 2000

Molecular biological analyses of in vitro aged CD4+ human T-cells

Medi ADIBZADEH, Andrea ENGEL and Graham PAWELEC
Tübingen Ageing and Tumour Immunology (TATI) Group, Section for Transplantation Immunology and Immunohaematology, Center for Medical Research of the University of Tübingen (ZMF), Waldhörnlestr. 22, D-72072 Tübingen, Germany

Abstract
Normal human CD4+ T cells have a finite life span in vitro and have been used as a model system for the study of in vivo aging. Altered patterns of gene expression may actively affect the T cell as it ages in vivo und in vitro. We have attempted to identify and analyse cDNA clones representing mRNAs differentially expressed between old and young T cell clones. We identified one cDNA (M213) which was isolated by subtractive techniques from a human T cell clone. Nucleotide sequence analysis of M213 cDNA clones revealed that they bore regions of homology to the human MHC II and CD1. Further, mRNA fingerprinting analysis of cells from old compared to young T cell clones implied that aging in vitro might be actively controlled by such changes in gene expression.

1. Introduction

Immunosenescence is defined as the deterioration of immune function in elderly individuals. As with other organ systems affected by ageing it occurs in animals and in humans. Observations that cellular lifespan is inversely proportional to the age of the cell donor *in vivo* and *in vitro,* as well as to the lifespan of the donor species, lend credence to the use of *in vitro* models of cellular ageing. However, more recent data cast some doubt on the general validity of this finding [1]. Transformation of normal human T cells (cultured *in vitro)* to an immortalized phenotype is an exceedingly rare event, although there may be limited examples of its occurrence, associated with the acquisition of striking chromosomal abnormalities [2]. We and others found that cultured human T cell clones always have limited lifespans [3-6].

There are two general theories for the causation of cellular senescence: first, the accumulation of mutations and DNA damage and increasingly inadequate repair mechanisms; second, the involvement of new genetic programmes actively regulating the lifespan. Cellular senescence may then result from a change in the balance of expression of positive growth regulatory genes along with the upregulation of inhibitory genes. Studies both in growth-arrested T-cells and in senescent fibroblasts suggest that the non-proliferative phenotype is actively maintained, since synthesis of new gene products is required. Induction of senescence in immortalized cell lines e.g. by chromosome transfer, further emphasized the dominant nature of proliferative "off" signals. For most of our cloned alloreactive $CD4^+$ helper T-cells, maintained in culture by intermittent restimulation with alloantigen in the presence of IL 2, a three-phase lifespan was shown with an entire finite lifespan extended up to a maximum of 60-80 population doublings (PD) on average. In phase I (up to ca. 35 estimated PD = "young"

TCC) T-cells can respond to antigen by autocrine IL 2-dependent clonal expansion. In phase II, they recognize antigen, but like T-cells of healthy elderly donors they show a specific defect in IL 2 production capacity and can no longer undergo autocrine proliferation; however, they continue to grow in the presence of exogenous growth factor. It is known further that these cells are characterized not only by loss of e.g. IL 2 secretion but by acquisition of other functional and structural properties. In phase III, they cease proliferating even in the presence of exogenous IL 2, senesce and die.

The molecular mechanisms underlying cellular senescence are not fully understood. When normal cells and immortal cells were fused, the resulting hybrids showed limited proliferative capacity [7]. Furthermore, when immortal cells were fused with each other, some combinations became mortal. By fusing immortal cells with each other, 21 human cell lines could be assigned to four complementation groups [8]. The same group observed that when mRNA fractions isolated from senescent human fibroblasts were microinjected into immortal cells, they inhibited DNA synthesis in proliferating cells [9]. These experiments suggest that the phenotype of finite division potential of human cells is dominant and that immortality results from recessive changes in the growth-regulation mechanisms of normal cells. All these data indicate that cellular senescence is a genetically programmed process. Several laboratories have attempted to find the gene or genes differentially expressed in senescent and young cells using various techniques. One hypothesis was, therefore, that it should be possible to isolate relevant genes by subtractive techniques ("old-minus-young"). In non-lymphoid cells, these strategies have to some extent been successful but studies on lymphocytes have not been reported so far and our intention here was the isolation of genes specifically upregulated in aged human T lymphocytes. In an attempt to design an experimental system which would enable us to distinguish between genes expressed in senescence as opposed to quiescence, cells from T cell clones (TCC) at an estimated one to three PD pre-senescence were stimulated with a CD3-specific monoclonal antibody together with IL 2 and then the RNA was isolated for use in a subtractive technique.

An alternative method that we describe for isolating genes of interest in old TCC in vitro is mRNA fingerprinting (DDRT-PCR; Differential Display Reverse Transcription Polymerase Chain Reaction) [10]. This method enables the identification of RNA which is expressed in one population, but absent in another, by using a set of arbitrary primers. Using this method it is possible to compare cells from old TCC with cells from the same young TCC in the same reaction and at the same time. This comparison is not possible using subtractive hybridisation. Further, this technique is simple, sensitive and requires only small amounts of RNA [10-13]. In the present report, we investigate the functional longevity of monoclonal human T lymphocytes as they progress from young to old populations in longitudinal studies and attempt to address the question of whether human T lymphocytes express senescence-specific genes which are not expressed in young proliferating cells.

2. Material and Methods

2.1 Cloning and propagation of T lymphocytes

Peripheral blood mononuclear cells (PBMC) isolated from a normal healthy donor were activated for 6 days in allogeneic MLC (mixed lymphocyte culture). Cells (2×10^6) were incubated in RPMI 1640 + 10% heat-inactivated pooled human nontransfused male serum with the same number of PBMC (20 Gy-irradiated) from an unrelated mismatched donor. After 6 days, cells were harvested and cloned by limiting dilution in the presence of highly purified natural IL 2 (Biotest Pharma, Dreieich, specific activity 2×10^7 U/mg). Lymphocyte populations from MLC with >75% blast cells were plated into Terasaki plates at 0.45, 4.5, and 45 cells per well again in the presence of the same irradiated PBMC, and in medium containing 16 % human serum and IL2. When more than 2/3 of the surface of a well was covered with growing cells, these were transferred to 7 diameter flat-bottomed microtiter plates with fresh medium, 1 x 10^5 Gy-irradiated B-LCL filler cells and IL 2. After a further 4-8 days, growing cells were again transferred to 16 diameter cluster plate wells with 2 x 10^5 B-LCL and maintained by subculturing every 7-10 days by splitting wells to 2 x 10^5 cloned cells per well and intermittently restimulating with alloantigen in the presence of IL 2 [14]. Cloning efficiencies were calculated from the number of cultures transferred to microtiter plates. Proliferative capacity of the clones was measured by assessing ^{3}H-thymidine incorporation. T cell-progenitors were obtained from PBMC by sorting the $CD7^+/CD3^-$ population and cloning as described [15, 16]. Briefly, PBMC were pre-incubated with human gamma globulin (Intraglobin, Biotest, Frankfurt) for 10 min and then double stained with monoclonal antibodies (mab) OKT3 (ATCC, CD3, IgG2a) and TÜ 93 (Tübingen local, CD7, IgG2b). After repeated washing the cells were incubated with goat anti-mouse IgG2a-PE and goat anti-mouse IgG2b-FITC (Southern Biotechnology). All steps were performed at 4°C. $CD7^+$ and $CD3^-$ cells were sorted three times on a FACS IV. An estimated enrichment factor of 30x yielded a calculated purity of >99.9% $CD7^+/CD3^-$ after 3 sorts.

2.2 Estimation of longevity

Terasaki wells which were scored as at least two-thirds full of growing cells were considered to contain a clone. The number of clones at this stage was used to calculate the average lifespan of the clones derived. The number of PD undergone was estimated from the multiplication factor at each cell count and subculture. The maximum lifespan was taken to be the time point of the death of the longest-living clone in each experiment.

2.3 Assessment of autocrine proliferation

1 x 10^4 cloned cells were incubated in triplicate with 80 Gy-irradiated B-lymphoblastoid cell lines (B-LCL) or stimulating agents in round-bottom microtiter plates for different periods of time, in RPMI medium supplemented with 10% human serum. Proliferation was quantified by measuring nuclear incorporation of tritiated thymidine (^{3}H-TdR, Amersham-Buchler, Braunschweig, specific activity 185 GBq/mmol used at 37 kBq/well) after a 14 h pulse label. Radioactivity was measured by liquid scintillation counting.

2.4 Reverse transcriptase-polymerase chain reaction (RT-PCR)

Total RNA was prepared using Isogen (Nippon Gene, Tokyo, Japan). One microgram of total RNA was reverse transcribed with 250 units of M-MLV reverse transcriptase (Gibco BRL, Karlsruhe) in 20 µl of reaction buffer containing 0.5 mM dNTP, 10 mM dithiothreitol, and 20 pmol of the oligo dT_{18} primer. After incubation at 42°C for 60 minutes, 3 µl of the reaction mixture was used for PCR. PCR was carried out with 0.5 units of Taq DNA polymerase (Pharmacia) in 50 µl of reaction buffer containing 0.25 mM dNTP, 20 pmol of each sense primer and antisense primer. Conditions for PCR were as follows: 94°C for 1 minute, 55°C for 1 minute, and 72°C for 2 minutes, for 35 cycles with a thermal cycler (Perkin Elmer, Norwalk, CT). The amplified products were subjected to electrophoresis on 1.5% agarose gels and visualized by ethidium bromide staining.

2.5 Primers.

Primers used for RT-PCR were synthesized by Pharmacia (Freiburg). Their sequences were as follows: ß-Actin sense, 5'-TGACGGGGTCACCCACACTGTGCCCATCTA-3` and antisense, 5'-CTAGAAGCATTGCGGTGGAGGATGGAGGG-3` [17]; Fas sense, 5'-GGAAGACTGTTACTACAGTTGAC-3', and antisense, 5'-GCCACTGTTTCAGGATTTAAGGTTGG -3' [18]; TGF-ß, sense, 5'-GTCACCCGCGTGCTAATGGTG -3', and antisense, 5'- CTCAATTTCCCCTCCACGGCT-3'; IL13, sense, 5'-GCATCCGCTCCTCAATCCTCT -3', and antisense, 5'-CGCGAGGGACGGTTCAACTGA-3' [19]. The predicted size of the fragment for ß-Actin is 661 base pairs (bp), for Fas, 540 bp, for IL13, 439 bp and for TGF-ß, 327 bp.

2.6 Construction and screening of the subtracted cDNA library.

An *in vitro* aged TCC (>55 days in culture up to a time corresponding to ca. 2 PD prior to senescence), stimulated overnight on OKT3-coated plates in the presence of IL 2, was taken as the source of mRNA for the synthesis of single stranded (ss) cDNA. Because of the large amount of mRNA (ca. 15-fold excess) needed for subtractive hybridization, it was not possible to take "young" cells from the same TCC. Therefore we isolated a pool of "young" T-cells from the same donor as that from which the "old" TCC was derived, using the "magnetic cell separation" (MACS) technique (Miltenyi Biotec GmbH). The cells were stained sequentially with OKT3, biotinylated goat anti-mouse moAb, fluorochrome-conjugated avidin, and superparamagnetic biotinylated microparticles, separated on high gradient magnetic columns, and controlled by FACS-analysis. These purified T-cells were also stimulated on OKT3 coated plates in the presence of IL 2

After cell lysis, total RNA was purified using $CsCl_2$-ultracentrifugation, and the mRNA separated over oligo(dT)-cellulose spin columns (Pharmacia, Freiburg). Before hybridizing, the template mRNA of the cDNA/mRNA-hybrid after first strand synthesis had to be removed with alkali. Then the synthesized ss cDNA of the old mRNA was hybridized in a high salt solution for 24-48 h at 68°C with an excess of photobiotinylated "young" mRNA. The resulting photobiotinylated ss cDNA"-"mRNA hybrids were complexed with free streptavidin and removed from the hybridization mixture by selective phenol/chloroform extraction (Subtraction-kit: Invitrogen Corp., ITC Biotechnology, Heidelberg). After a second purification step using a water-jacketed hydroxylapatite column (HTP grade, Bio-Rad) maintained at 55-60°C, the unbound ss cDNA was pure enough to serve as a hybridization probe or for establishing a subtracted cDNA library after second strand synthesis. We ligated the blunt-ended ds cDNA to a Sma I-cut pUC13 vector and transformed competent E. coli DH5α. Colony- and plasmid-blots were then hybridized differentially with cDNA probes made from "old" TCC and "young" T-cells. A flow chart of this subtractive technique is shown in Fig. 1.

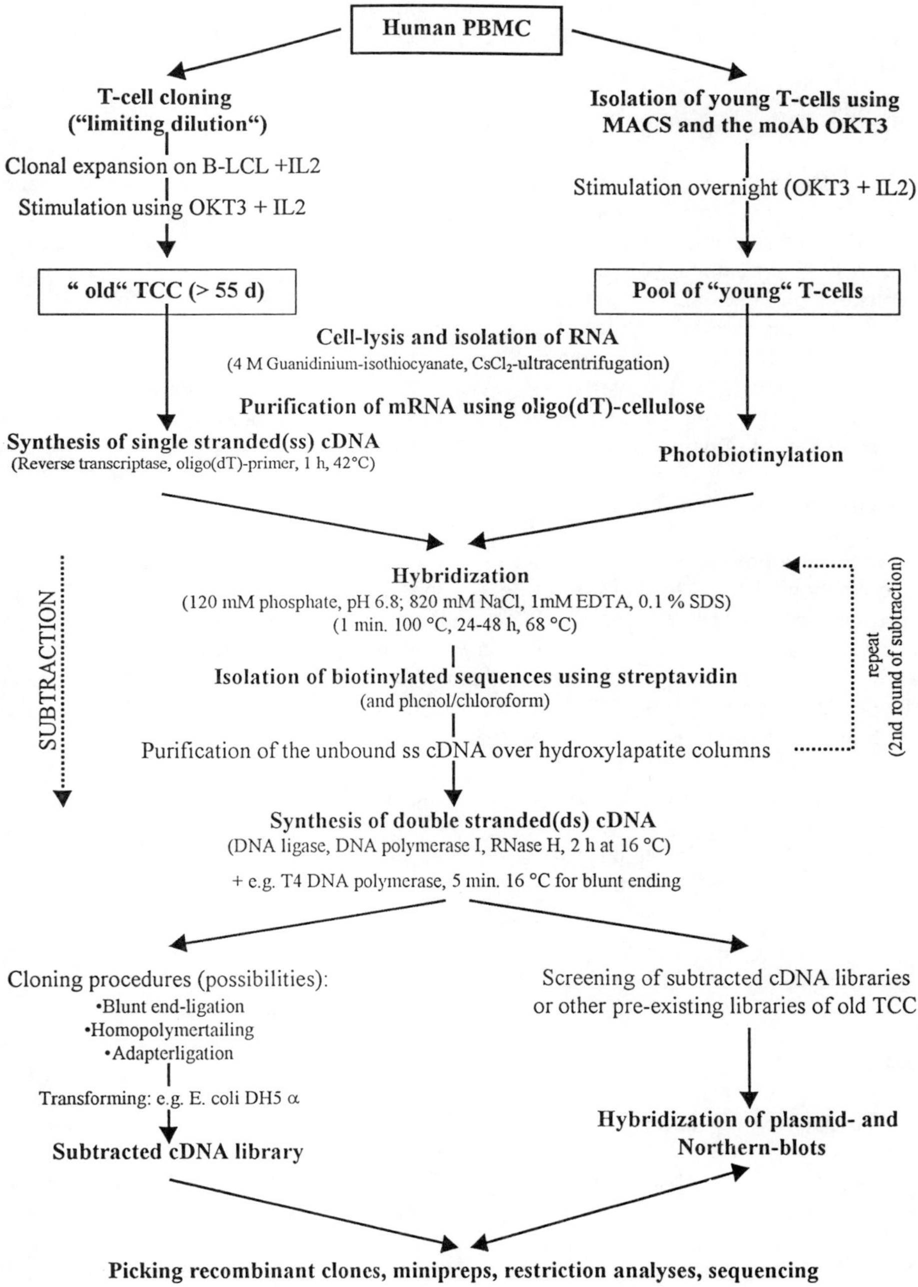

Fig. 1. The method of subtractive cDNA library construction.

2.7 DNA-Sequencing:

Double-stranded plasmid DNA was directly sequenced following the dideoxy chain termination method of Sanger et al. [20]. The sequence data were analysed with the Genius/Husar-system (DKFZ, Heidelberg) and compared with EMBL or GenBank data base sequences.

2.8 mRNA fingerprinting

1µg of total RNA or 100 ng of poly$(A)^+$ RNA was added to a sterile microcentrifuge tube. The total volume was adjusted to 14.5 µl with DEPC-treated water to which 1 µl of the 25 µM arbitrary primer stock was added. The reaction was incubated for 10 minutes at 70°C, then chilled for 1 minute on ice and the contents collected by brief centrifugation. Following centrifugation, reagents were added as follows: 2 µl of 10x first-strand buffer, 1 µl of RNase Block Ribonuclease Inhibitor (40 U/µl), 1 µl of dNTP mix (25 mM each NTP) and 0.5 µl of MMLV-RT (50 U/µl). The contents were gently mixed and collected by brief centrifugation in a microcentrifuge. Incubation followed at room temperature for 10 minutes, then 60 minutes at 37°C. Then the reaction was heated to 90°C for 5 minutes to inactivate the reverse transcriptase, and finally chilled on ice for 10 minutes.

2.9 Polymerase Chain Reaction

The following components were added to a sterile microcentrifuge tube. 5 µl of 10x Taq reaction buffer, 0.4 µl of dNTP mix (25 mM each NTP), 3 µl of 25 mM $MgCl_2$ (3 mM final concentration), 0.2 µl of Taq DNA polymerase (5 U/µl), 2 µl of the 25 mM arbitrary primer stock, and 10 µl of a 1: 10 dilution of cDNA. The total volume was adjusted to 50 µl with DEPC-treated water and. gently mixed, then collected the bottom of microcentrifuge tube by brief centrifugation. RT-PCR was performed using the cycling conditions outlined in the following table:

Number of cycles	Length of time	Temperature
1 cycle	5 minutes	94°C
	5 minutes	60°C
40 cycles	2 minutes	72°C
	1 minute	94°C
	1 minute	60°C
1 cycle	10 minutes	72°C

3. Results

3.1 The cloning efficiency

To clarify whether aging in vivo has any effect on the cloning efficiency of stimulated T cells, peripheral blood mononuclear cells (PBMC) were isolated from young (19, 20, and 22 years) and older (59, 60, 65, and 72 years) healthy donors. The cells were stimulated and cloned by limiting dilution. The Terasaki wells which were two-thirds or completely full of growing cells were designated positive and the percentage of the positive wells was used to calculate the cloning efficiencies (CE, Table 1). The average CE of the young donors was 33.5% and of the old donors 32%. In this experiment the CE between young and old healthy donors was surprisingly similar. However, further culture of cells derived from old donors proved to be impossible.

	CE %	Average CE %
PBMC isolated from young healthy donors	19 years old 30% 20 years old 34% 22 years old (a) 37% 22 years old (b) 33%	33.5%
PBMC isolated from old healthy donors	59 years old 31% 60 years old 34% 65 years old 31% 72 years old 32%	32%

Table 1. The cloning efficiencies of young and old donors.

3.2 Cell growth

As an example of the growth kinetics of the TCC examined, growth curves of three clones from younger donors are shown in Fig. 2. Cumulative cell number per clone is shown at the different culture time points indicated after intermittent restimulation of a starting number of cells of 2 x 10^6 (Fig. 2). The number of TCC 4-56 and 13-8 cells increased up to culture day 43 - 50, and then decreased with further time in culture. In the case of TCC 4-8, the cell number was practically constant and the T cell clone divided slowly and died after 71 days.

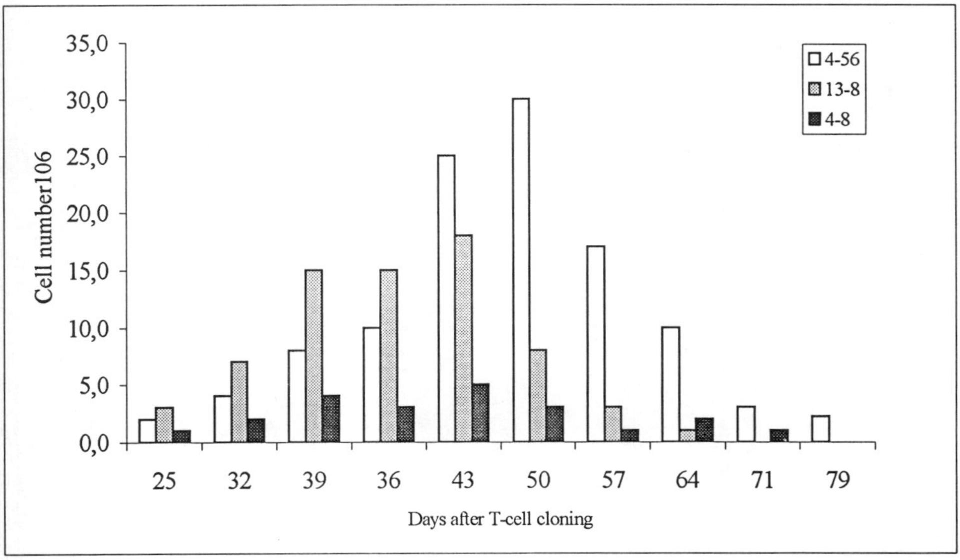

Fig. 2. Cell growth at different times after T-cell cloning. The cumulative cell number of three TCC, starting with 2 x 10^6, was determined at each time point.

3.3 Proliferative capacity of young and old TCC

To investigate whether the growth rate of TCC is related to autocrine proliferative capacity of TCC, we measured thymidine incorporation of young and old cells from three different allospecific TCC. The old TCC are defined as being 2 PD before senescence. In Fig. 3 we confirm that senescent TCC 13-29, 49-59, and 49-65 lost their autocrine proliferative capacity after culture in vitro. These T cell clones senescensed and could not further proliferate in the presence of APC.

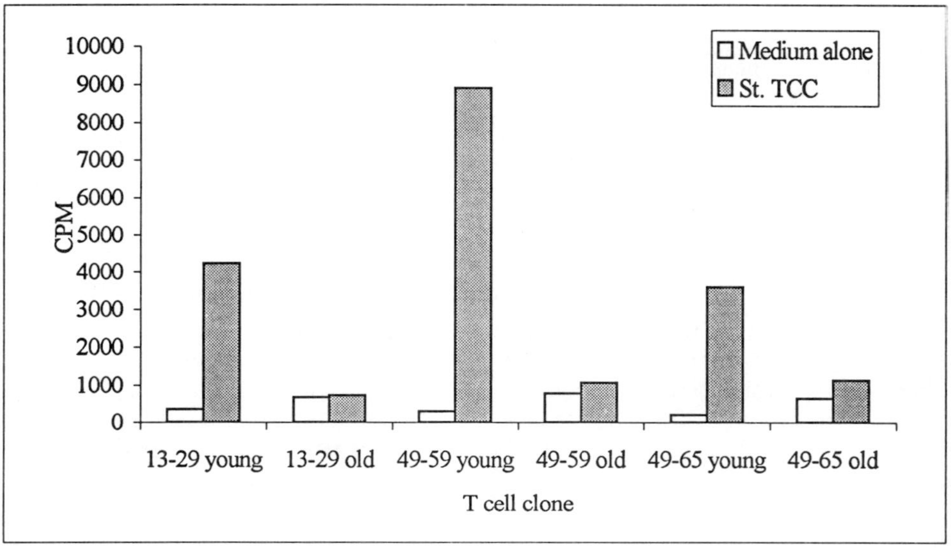

Fig. 3. Proliferative capacity of young and old TCC.

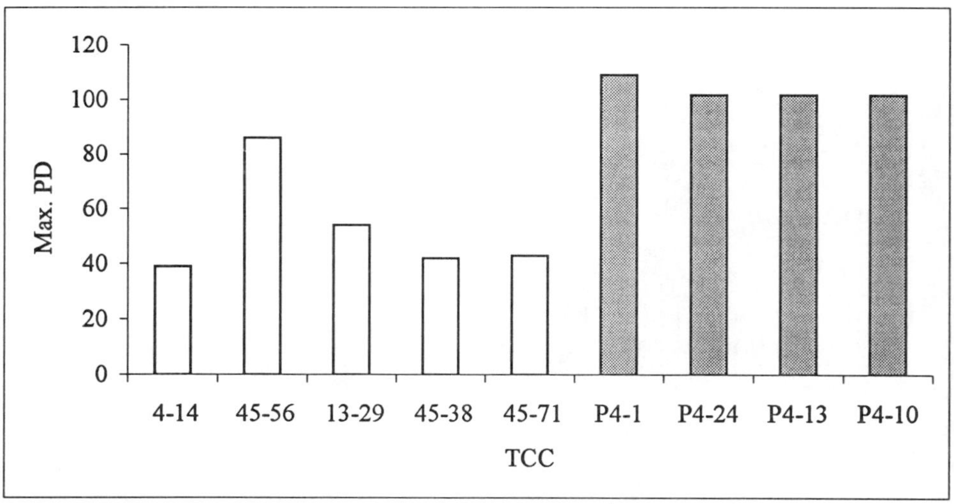

Fig. 4. The lifespans of five TCC from PBMC and four TCC from $CD7^+/CD3^-$ progenitor T-cells.

3.4 Maximum lifespan of TCC

The lifespans of five TCC derived from PBMC and four TCC from $CD7^+/CD3^-$ progenitor T-cells are shown in Fig. 4. The lifespan of PBMC-derived TCC 4-14, 45-38, and 45-71 TCC was about 40 PD, and of 4-56 and 13-29 was somewhat greater. The average here was 52.8

PD, whereas the average lifespan of the four $CD7^{+}/CD3^{-}$negative-derived TCC was 103.75 PD. This difference between the maximum lifespans of TCC derived from PBMC (52,8 PD) and TCC from CD7+/CD3- progenitor T-cells (103,75) may reflect (represent) the length of time required for the pre T cells to develop into mature T cells in vitro.

3.5 PCR-analysis in old and young TCC

Possible reasons for lack of proliferation of old T cell clones might have involved increased TGF-ß cytokine secretion, or increased susceptibility of the CD95 (fas)-positive T cells to killing by Fas-Ligand. We therefore analysed accumulated mRNA for TGF-ß and Fas by PCR in an old and a young TCC (Fig. 5.). The mRNA expression of TGF-ß and Fas is positive in the old but not in the young TCC. The expression of IL 13 ,which is very important for the regulation of inflammatory and immune responses, decreased in the old TCC in comparison to the young TCC. Stimulated PBMC were used as positive controls.

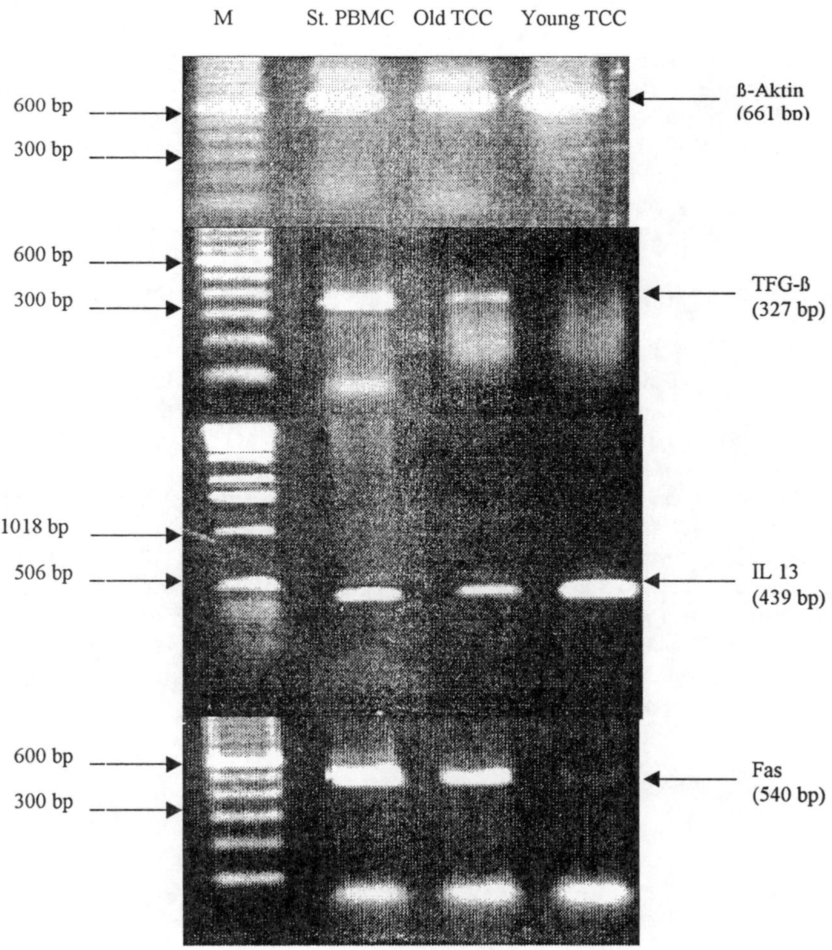

Fig. 5. PCR-analysis in old and young TCC.

3.6 Subtractive hybridization

For isolating gene candidates from *in vitro* aged TCC, possibly regulating the process of cellular senescence, we established an efficient subtractive method. More than 1200 clones of the subtracted cDNA library were again screened for hybridization to random primer labeled ds cDNA from "old" and "young" TCC. Fig. 6 shows one of these hybridization results and also our problems with background using these probes even under highly stringent conditions (using the method of Church and Gilbert) [21]. One clone (*) with a ca. 300 bp insert (pM213) reacts only with the cDNA probe of the "old" TCC and preliminary Northern blot analysis revealed further that this gene sequence seems to be preferentially expressed in "old" TCC but to a lesser extent also in certain "young" TCC. Analysing the sequence revealed a high percentage of identity to CD1 (thymocyte antigen, 72% of 196bp overlap) and MHC (major histocompatibility complex) class II genes (70-80% of ca. 110-150bp overlap). Unfortunately, the insert contains part of an intron region with a small repeat and is therefore responsible for the relatively high background when used as a hybridization probe in Northern- and Southern-blot analyses (Fig. 7), and presumably for the high percentage of identity to MHC-like genes. In further experiments we used the whole 300 bp insert and also specific oligonucleotides flanking the repeat for screening again both the starting subtracted cDNA library and a complete cDNA library established from an "old" TCC in PSPORT (Gibco, BRL) to isolate clones with inserts containing longer coding regions. 12 new sequences (500-3000bp), which have mostly retained their hybridization pattern, could be identified and some of these were partly sequenced. Currently, sequencing data show no notable homologies to any other EMBL or GenBank sequences.

3.7 Differential Display Reverse Transcription Polymerase Chain Reaction

One problem with the subtractive hybridization was that insufficient RNA was available from each TCC to use for the subtractive hybridisation and for the quantification of gene expression in old and young TCC. An alternative technique is the Differential Display Reverse Transcription Polymerase Chain Reaction (DDRT-PCR). This method is based on the reverse transcription of RNA and the amplification of cDNA with a set of arbitrary primers.

DDRT-PCR uses combinations of 10-mer arbitrary primers with anchored cDNA primers and generates fragments that originate mostly from the poly-A^+ tail and extend about 50-600 nucleotides upstream [10-13]. The original differential display (DDRT-PCR) technique [10, 12] should be able to generate a largely complete pattern of all mRNAs expressed in a particular cell using a reasonable number of primer pairs [12]. In this technique, cDNA is amplified in a PCR with low-stringency annealing (at 42~C) throughout. The PCR primers consist of 10-base arbitrary primer and the same locking primer used in the first strand synthesis ($T_{11}VN$; V can be A,G or C, N can be any of the four nucleotides).

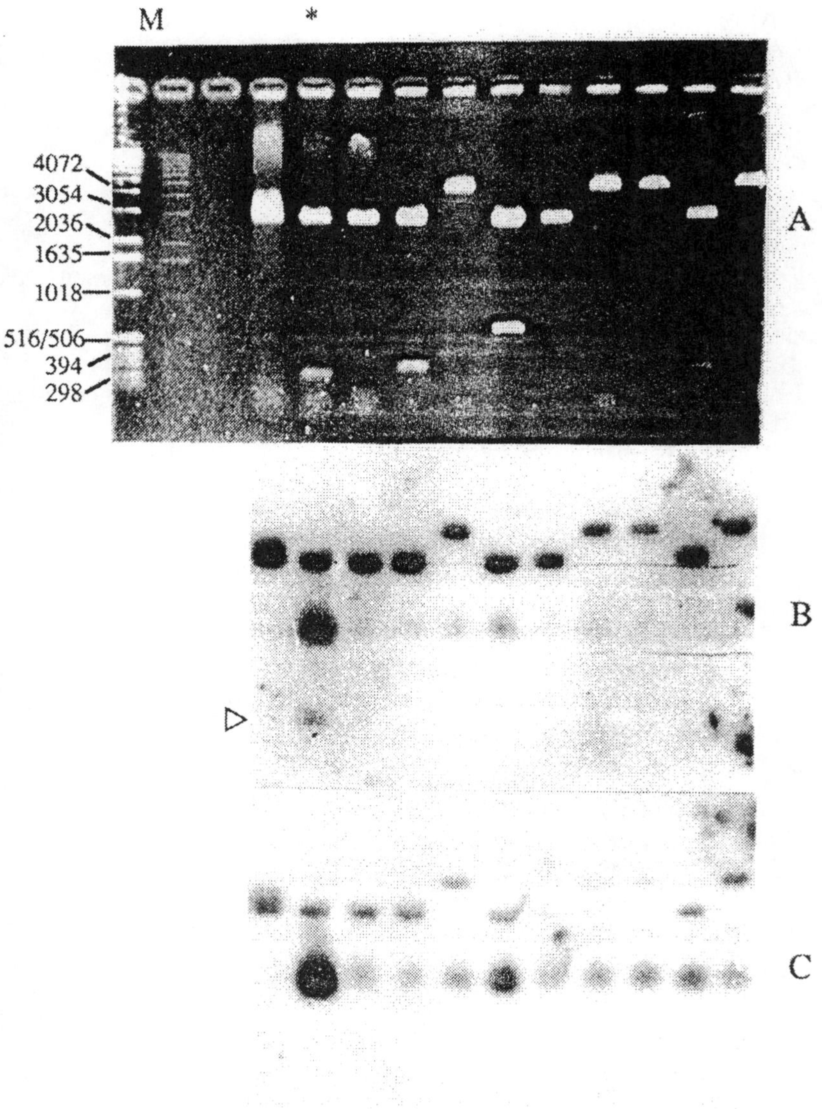

Fig. 6. Subtractive hybridization: A) EcoRI x BamHI-restriction of some randomly picked recombinant pUC13 clones of the subtracted cDNA library, *: pM213 (ca. 300 bp insert). B) Southern-blot analyses using cDNA established from an in vitro aged TCC (2 PD before senescence), stimulated with OKT 3 and C) cDNA established from young stimulated T-cells of the same donor as hybridization probes.

5`- AAC ACT ACA CAC GAA AGT AGA GTG TCT CAA GTT GTA AAG AAA ACT AAC TCG TCA ACC CTT TGT CAG ACA AAC ACC TTA GAC GTT TCC ATA AAA AAA AGA ATA AAA AAT AAA TAA AAA TAA AAA TAA AAA TAA AAT AAT AAT AAT ATG AAA TTC AAA ATC TCA-3`

Fig. 7. Nucleotide sequence of pM213.

The process of the DDRT-PCR is the following:

1) During the first strand synthesis, the locking primer samples a sizeable portion of the mRNA (potentially 1/16th) present in the cell.
2) The arbitrary primer permits amplification of reverse-transcribed cDNA species using the locking primer.
3) Repeated PCR cycling with low stringency results in amplification of products of a size <500bp that can be evaluated on standard acrylamide-gels.

Fig.8. Shows DDRT-PCR analysis of four old and four young stimulated TCC. Two fragments (φ) with a ca. 170bp and 910bp were amplified only in old TCC but not by young TCC. These DNA fragments were isolated from a gel, re-amplified and transfered to a membrane for slot blot analysis (Fig. 9).

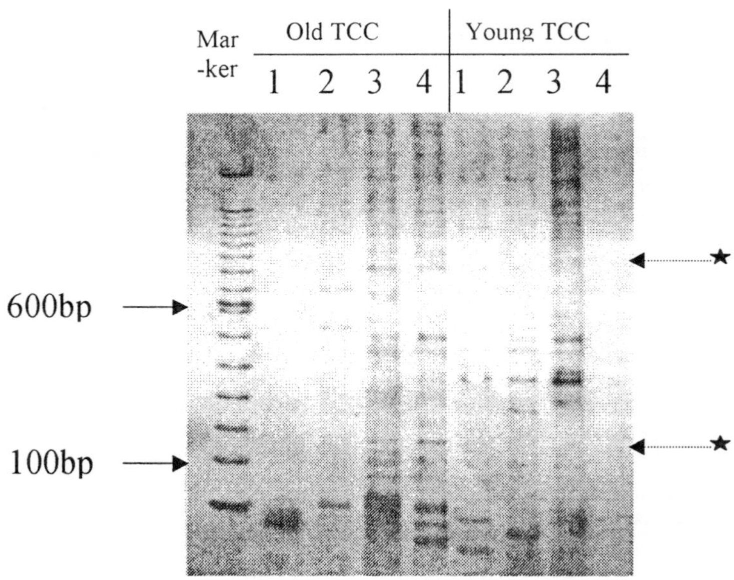

Fig. 8. DDRT-PCR analysis of four old and four young stimulated T cell clones. Two fragments (φ) with a ca. 170bp and 910bp were expressed only in old TCC.

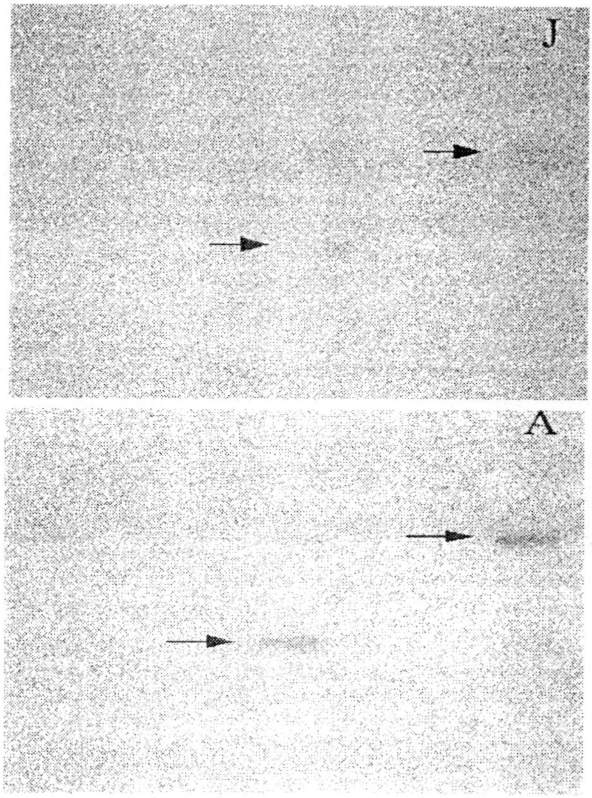

Fig. 9. Shows the autoradiograph of slot blot hybridization using dscDNA from the old TCC (A) and young TCC (J). This slot blot analysis confirms the upregulation of the genes in old TCC clones.

The Slot blot analysis confirms the upregulation of genes in old (A) T cell clones but not in young (J) T cell clones (Fig. 9).

4. Discussion

More than 30 years ago, Hayflick reported that diploid fibroblasts undergo a finite number of cell divisions, after which they stop proliferating. This phenomenon was termed replicative senescence [22]. Later it was found that other cell types undergo replicative senescence, including smooth-muscle cells, melanocytes, and T lymphocytes [6, 23, 24]. In this study we have attempted to establish a model for clonal ageing of T cells using long-term in vitro cultures, observing their altered characteristics over time. Further we have attempted to address the question of whether old human T lymphocytes express senescence-specific genes, which are not expressed in young T cells.

It is well established that the majority of elderly individuals manifest depressed T lymphocyte function in a variety of in vitro and in vivo assays. We compared here the cloning efficiencies of T cells from young and old healthy donors and found that while they were comparable, establishment of long-term clones was not possible from the latter. We confirmed that the longevity of T cell clones derived in vitro from T cell progenitors was approximately 104 PD, which is greater than for T cell clones derived from mature peripheral T cells under these particular culture conditions [25]. The reason for the increase of PD by CD3-/CD7+ population may be that the "clock" is first switched on at the time point when the progenitor becomes a fully differentiated mature T cell.

The work reported here attempted to address the question of whether human T lymphocytes express senescence-specific genes not expressed in "young" proliferating cells. In order to increase the likelihood of obtaining senescent- and not quiescent-related sequences, both T-cell populations for our novel subtractive technique were stimulated with the CD3 moAb prior to isolating mRNA. Preliminary results from these difficult experiments have in fact provided some evidence for at least one sequence, designated pM213, which may be a candidate for such senescence-associated genes. It hybridized only with a labeled cDNA probe from "old" but not "young" TCC of the same donor. The sequence of this pM213 insert showed most significant homology to CD1 and MHC class II genes (70-80% over up to 200bp). The sequence homologies with MHC-related genes are interesting in the light of structural and functional data we have obtained earlier on the expression of putative novel MHC products by aged $CD4^+$ human helper TCC. Sequential immunoprecipitation experiments with TCC > ca. 35 PD (phase II) suggested that the upregulated MHC class II-like molecules differ from all known classical class II and class II-like molecules [26]. Other short fragments obtained showed some homology to insulin-like growth factor 1, p53, other class II genes and K-ras. Nevertheless, all of these homologies were over limited stretches and their significance remains in doubt.

Alternative techniques to subtractive hybridization are the differential display reverse transcription polymerase chain reaction [10] and RNA arbitrarily primed polymerase chain reaction (RAP-PCR) [27]. Both techniques provide a simple and reproducible method for fingerprinting mRNA transcripts. In DDRT-PCR the cDNA is amplified in a PCR with low-stringency annealing temperature (42°C) throughout, whereas in RAP-PCR 18-mer arbitrary primers allow high-stringency PCR amplification and minimal chance of amplifying genomic DNA. The PCR consists of a single round of low-stringency amplification followed by multiple rounds with higher stringency. At the beginning of our study we started with the method of DDRT-PCR and obtained PCR products of up to 500 bp. In this case we were not able to reamplify the PCR products under low-stringency PCR conditions. For further experiments we used Oligo`s dT_{18} cDNA as a first strand and amplified with 18-mer arbitrary primers. In this system, PCR products of greater than 500bp could be obtained after high-stringency PCR amplification.

Acknowledgements

It was a great pleasure to work with all the researchers of the EUCAMBIS group. This work was performed under the aegis of the European Union Concerted Action on the Molecular Biology of Immunosenescence EUCAMBIS (contract BMHI-CT94-1209) and partially supported by grants from the Deutsche Forschungsgemeinschaft (DFG).

5. References

[1] V.J. Cristofalo, R.G. Allen, R.J. Pignolo, B.G. Martin and J.C. Beck, Relationship between donor age and the replicative lifespan of human cells in culture: A reevaluation. Proc. Natl. Acad. Sci. USA **95** (1998) 10614-10619.

[2] K. Kaltoft, C.B. Pedersen, B.H. Hansen and K. Thestrup-Pedersen, Appearance of isochromosome 18q can be associated with in vitro immortalization of human T lymphocytes. Cancer Genet. Cytogenet. **81** (1995) 13-16.

[3] M. McCarron, Y. Osborne, C. Story, J.L. Dempsey, R. Turner and A. Morley, Effect of age on lymphocyte proliferation. Mech. Ageing Dev. **41** (1987) 211-218.

[4] R.B. Effros and R.L. Walford, Neonatal T cells as a model system to study the possible in vitro senescence of lymphocytes. Exp. Gerontol. **22** (1987) 307-316.

[5] R.B. Effros, Decline in CD28(+) T cells in centenarians and in long-term T cell cultures: a possible cause for both in vivo and in vitro immunosenescence. Exp. Gerontol. **29** (1994) 601-609.

[6] N.L. Perillo, R.L. Walford, M.A. Newman and R.B. Effros, Human T lymphocytes possess a limited in vitro lifespan. Exp. Gerontol. **24** (1989) 177-187.

[7] G.H. Stein and R.M. Yanishevsky, Entry into S phase is inhibited in two immortal cell lines fused to senescent human diploid cells, Exp. Cell Res. **120** (1979) 155-165.

[8] O.M. Pereira-Smith and J.R. Smith, Genetic analysis of indefinite division in human cells: Identification of four complemention groups, Proc. Natl. Acad. Sci. USA **85** (1988) 6042-6046.

[9] C.K. Jr. Lumpkin, J.K. McClung, O.M. Pereira-Smith and J.R. Smith, Existence of high abundance antiproliferative mRNAs in senescent human diploid fibroblasts. Science **232** (1986) 393-395.

[10] P. Liang and A.B. Pardee, Differential display of eukaryotic messenger RNA by means of the polymerase chain reaction. Science **257** (1992) 967-971.

[11] D. Bauer, H. Muller, J. Reich, V. Ahrenkiel, P. Warthoe and M. Strauss, Identification of differentially expressed mRNA species by an improved display technique (DDRT-PCR). Nucleic Acids Res. **21** (1993) 4272-4280.

[12] P. Liang, L. Averboukh and A.B. Pardee, Distribution and cloning of eukaryotic mRNAs by rneans of differential display: refinements and optimization. Nucleic Acids Res. **21** (1993) 3269-3275.

[13] J.W. Zimmermann and R.M. Schultz, Analysis of gene expression in the preimplantation mouse embryo: use of mRNA differential display. Proc. Natl. Acad. Sci. USA **91** (1994) 5456-5460.

[14] G. Pawelec, Cloning and propagation of human T lymphocytes. In G. Gallagher, R.C. Rees and C.W. Reynolds (eds.), Tumour Immunobiology. A Practical Approach. IRL Press, Oxford (1993) 131-141.

[15] H. Pohla, M. Adibzadeh, H.J. Bühring, et al., Evolution of a CD3+ CD4+ alpha/beta T-cell receptor-positive mature T cell clone from CD3-/CD7+ sorted human bone marrow cells. Dev. Immunol. **3** (1993) 197-210.

[16] M. Adibzadeh, H.J. Buhring, T. Daikeler, P. Siegels-Hübenthal, M. Owsianowsky, A. Schenk, A. Rehbein, K. Schaudt, E. Schlotz, H. Pohla and G. Pawelec, Extrathymic Development and Function of Human T-Lymphocytes from Bone Marrow Cells in Vitro. Cell. Immunol. **154** (1994) 25-42.

[17] S. Ehlers and K.A. Smith, Differentiation of T-cell lymphokine gene expression: The in vitro acquisition of T cell memory. J. Exp. Med. 173 (1991) 25-36.

[18] N. Itoh, S. Yonehara, A. Ishii, M. Yonehara, S.I. Mizushima, M. Sameshima, A. Hase, Y. Seto and S. Nagata, The polypeptide encoded by the cDNA for human cell surface antigen Fas can mediate apoptosis. Cell **66** (1991) 233-243.

[19] A. Minty, P. Chalon, J.M. Derocq, X. Dumont, J.C. Guillemot, M. Kaghad, C. Labit, P. Leplatois, P. Liauzun and B. Miloux, Interleukin-13 is a new human lymphokine regulating inflammatory and immune responses. Nature **362** (1993) 248-250.

[20] F. Sanger, S. Nicklen and A.R. Coulson, DNA sequencing with chain-terminating inhibitors. Proc. Natl. Acad. Sci. USA **74** (1977) 5463-5467.

[21] G.M. Church and W. Gilbert, Genomic sequencing. Proc. Natl. Acad. Sci. USA **81** (1984) 1991-1995.

[22] L. Hayflick, The limited in vitro lifetime of human diploid cell strains. Exp. Cell Res. **37** (1965) 614-636.

[23] G. Pawelec, P. Wernet, A. Rehbein, I. Balko and E.M. Schneider, Alloproliferative human T cell clones primed and cultured in vitro lose proliferative and gain suppressive activity with age. Human Immunology **10** (1984) 135-142.

[24] R.B. Effros, Replicative senescence in the immune system: impact of the Hayflick limit on T-cell function in the elderly. Am. J. Hum. Gene. **62** (1998) 1003-1007.

[25] M. Adibzadeh, H. Pohla, A. Rehbein and G. Pawelec, Long-term culture of monoclonal human T lymphocytes: models for immunosenescence? Mech. Ageing Dev. **83** (1995) 171-183.

[26] G. Pawelec, N. Fernandez, T. Brocker, E.M. Schneider, H. Festenstein and P. Wernet, DY determinants, possibly associated with novel class II molecules, stimulate autoreactive $CD4^+$ T cells with suppressive activity. J. Exp. Med. **167** (1988) 243-261.

[27] J. Welsh, K. Chada, S.S. Dalal, R. Cheng, D. Ralph and M. McClelland, Arbitrarily primed PCR fingerprinting of RNA. Nucleic Acids

EUCAMBIS: Immunology and Ageing in Europe
G. Pawelec (Ed.)
IOS Press, 2000

Aging of the Immune System

Carlo Bartoloni, Luisa Guidi, Augusto Tricerri, Andrea Riccardo Errani, Mario Costanzo, *Gino Doria, *Daniela Frasca
*Institute of Internal Medicine and Geriatrics, Catholic University, Largo A. Gemelli 8, 00168, Rome and *Laboratory of Immunology, ENEA CR Casaccia, V. Anguillarese 301, 00060 Rome (Italy)*

Abstract
During senescence, alterations of the immune system affect both antibody and cell-mediated responses. Virgin cells are replaced by memory cells, cells with signal transduction defects accumulate and the profile of Th1 and Th2 cytokines changes. These modifications may produce suitable conditions for T cell-mediated dysregulation of antibody responses characterized by the production of low affinity and self-reactive antibodies. Moreover, the response of naive T cells from old subjects and, to a lesser extent, of naive and memory T cells from young subjects to CD3 cross-linking can be augmented by the addition of IL-2 and IL-12. These results underscore the potential use of cytokines as adjuvants in vaccination.

1. Introduction

Aging is a process that changes healthy individuals into weak ones, with decreased performance of most physiological systems and increased susceptibility to disease and death. All disabilities, including declines in cardiovascular and neurosensory functions, immune responsiveness, and resistance to neoplastic and degenerative disease, display similar patterns in all mammalian species and affect the mean life span. Conversely, the rate of aging, as expressed by the maximum life span potential (life span of the longest-lived member of a very large population), varies across species in mammals over a 30 fold range, from 3 years in rodent to >120 years in humans. The mean life span, which is influenced by illness, has been greatly enhanced in humans since antiquity, owing to the improvements in public healthy conditions. However, on the average, people live longer today but still age at the same rate as in the past, for the age of the longest-lived survivor has remained the same not only irrespective of place out but even since ancient times [1].

2. Genes and aging

The aging rate is under genetic control, as supported by the following considerations. a) All animal species have characteristic rates of aging. b) The progeny of animals from two inbred strains have life spans longer than those of either parental strain (heterosis). c) In humans, females live longer than males as in most animal species. It is opposite, however, in some mouse and rat strains. d) Parents who die at ages beyond the average life expectancy have children who are more likely to leave longer as well.

It should be stresses, however, that non-genetic factors may also play a role in generating the impairments that lead to manifestations of aging. The cross-linking of collagen may be a kind of change that occurs over time and that is probably not directly influenced by a genetic program and yet might contribute to senescence changes. Thus, at the level of macromolecules, their stability may not require a genetic basis. The accumulation of lipofuscin and the denaturation of organelles and enzyme molecules having regular turnover rates may represent other examples of molecular changes occurring over time that do not necessarily require genetic information. Other non-genetic mechanisms are endocrine and neural factors which appear to regulate age changes in target cells. It should be pointed out, however, that the genetic control of these factors has not been ruled out. [2].

The genetic control of the aging rate makes stochastic processes due to random events unlikely [3] and favours programmed events encoded in part of the genome, as a master clock, and expressed as a molecular mechanism accounting for the synchrony of structural and functional changes in different cells and tissues of each member of a given species [4, 5]. Identification of the genes and processes that set the aging rate differently in different species has been attempted by several approaches.

A limited gene theory of aging [6] has considered the role of the MHC that controls immunoregulatory cell functions and interactions. Furthermore, genes within the MHC together with other MHC-related genes regulating superoxide dismutase, mixed function oxidase, and the level of cyclic nucleotides have been postulated to constitute a multigene family exerting a multifactorial influence on the aging process [7]. Besides affecting immune functions, this multigene family appears to regulate enzymes protecting against free radical-induced damage, which accumulates in aging [8], as well as cyclic nucleotides involved in cell proliferation and differentiation, which show marked age-related alterations [9]. Experiments with congenic mice [6] have shown that although genetically identical except for the short MHC region, the mice within each set display considerable variation in maximum life span. However, evidence was provided for a complex interaction between a particular allele and the over-all genetic background as a single allele promotes either longer or shorter life span depending upon the several backgrounds.

3. DNA repair and aging

Using congenic mice it has also been shown that the MHC influences the DNA repair capacity [10], a property which is positively correlated with the maximum life span in several mammalian species [11]. The role of DNA repair in cellular aging has recently raised great interest following the identification of cellular proteins that play a key role in DNA damage recognition and repair pathways [12]. The damage is firstly recognized by nuclear proteins displaying helicase activity, and the DNA repair is than carried out under the control of other proteins. In eukariotic cells, the repair of DNA double strand breaks proceeds in a number of different steps, each of which is under the control of specific proteins with distinct biochemical and functional properties. Briefly, after the recognition of the damage by helicases, an endonuclease initiates the DNA excision-repair by making incisions upstream of the strand break. Then an exonuclease remove a short oligonucleotide containing the strand break, creating a gapped duplex. A DNA repair polymerase fills the gap and a DNA ligase seals the replaced DNA segment to complete the repair process [reviewed in 13]. Eukaryotic cells contain many copies of the helicase ku 70/80 protein. This protein has been reported to be involved in the control of DNA replication and transcription and in V(D)J recombination. Ku 80-deficient mice exhibit severe combined immunodeficiency due to T and B lymphocyte arrest at early progenitor stages. Ku is able to bind not only to DNA ends, but also to other alterations in double-stranded DNA, such as hairpins, nicks and gaps. Ku has also been reported to bind to other enzymes of the repair cascade, such as DNA ligase III. Furthermore, ku is the DNA binding component of a DNA-dependent protein kinase (DNA-PK) which can phosphorylate a wide range of nuclear factors. The ability of ku to recognize and bind to double strand DNA ends suggests that its binding could represent an early step in the repair process. The functional substrates of the phosphorylation have only been in part identified but could include components of the transcription or replication machinery to arrest their action, or proteins involved directly in the repair process itself. Alternatively the large DNA-PK complex could hold DNA ends in a configuration promoting their rejoining. DNA-PK might also regulate the assembly of multiprotein complexes or, alternatively, it might act more indirectly by regulating the expression of genes that are involved in the repair process or in a linked process, such as cell cycle regulation. This latter function of the DNA-PK would provide an effective mechanism able to block DNA replication before cells have repaired their damaged DNA.

We have recently investigated the relationship between the helicase ku protein, involved in the earliest steps of double-stranded DNA break recognition, and the mitotic responsiveness in aging. Our results from a survey of human populations of different ages (26-95 years) have shown that PBL from all elderly subjects (65-95 years) display low mitotic responses to PHA but only a limited number exhibit reduced amounts of ku 70/80, suggesting that age-related impairment in DNA repair is only marginally related to reduced expression of ku protein. As discussed elsewhere [14], either a higher frequency of DNA breaks is required for evident activation of repair processes or other steps of the cascade of events are more compromised than ku protein helicase activity in aging. In line with this observation, we have observed significant differences in the DNA-binding activity of the heterodimer ku 70/80 when PBL from subjects of different ages were *in vitro* irradiated with the sublethal dose of 500 cGy of X-rays, the DNA-binding activity of the ku protein being 10-15-fold enhanced by X-rays in PBL from young subjects, whereas it was unchanged in irradiated PBL from elderly subjects [15].

4. Aging of cells of the immune system

Aging is characterized by decreased humoral and cell mediated immunity to a large variety of exogenous antigens and by an increased propensity to autoimmune phenomena, suggesting an age-related dysregulation of the immune system [16-19]. Alterations in cellular components of the immune system rather than in the extracellular *milieu* accounts for most of the variations of the immune response with aging [20]. The decrease in immune reactivity with increasing age may reflect multiple events, affecting cell proliferation and differentiation, leading to reduction in cell number and function within immune cell populations [21].

Stem cells, the progenitors of lymphocytes and accessory cells, have been thoroughly investigated to detect changes in their proliferative and differentiative capacities, and found in most studies to be unimpaired by aging [22, 24]. However, when competitive repopulation assays were used to detect subtle effects of aging on bone marrow stem cell to colonize the thymic stroma, marrow from older mice was found to be less able to initiate thymocyte maturation after *in vitro* transfer to a young thymic environment. Results from limiting dilution assays suggest an age-related decrease of prothymocyte frequency in the bone marrow [25]. A recent survey on aging humans has also indicated reduced numbers of committed hematopoietic progenitor cells, as indicated by surface markers and functions [26].

Age influences both antibody and cell-mediated immune response, T cell responses being more severely affected than B cell responses. T cell proliferative responses to antigens and mitogens and T cell-mediate responses such as cutaneous delayed-type hypersensitivity, mixed lymphocyte reactivity, and cell mediated cytotoxicity, decreased with aging [27]. Precursor frequency analysis of T cells, by limiting dilution techniques, indicates that the fraction of responding T cell precursors declines with aging, but the progeny of each cell precursor maintains full proliferative capacity and immunocompetence [28].

Aging negatively affects the membrane structures involved in the early events of T cell activation [29, 30] (Tables 1 and 2)

Table 1

Effect of aging on membrane structures of murine T cells

Membrane structures	Resting T cells	Activated T cells
Thy 1	no effect	
CD3	no effect	
TCR α/β	no effect	
CD4/CD8	decrease	
CD28	slight increase	decrease
CTLA-4	increase	decrease
IL-2αβγ		decrease
CD95 (Fas)	no effect	decrease
L-selectin	decrease	
$R123^{lo}$ ($P\text{-}Gly^{-}$ cells)		decrease
$R123^{hi}$ ($P\text{-}Gly^{+}$ cells)		decrease

T cells from aged mice exhibit defects in calcium mobilization [31-34] and protein phosphorylation due to both tyrosine-specific [35, 36] and serine-, threonine-specific [37] kinases, which lead to changes in signal transduction pathways. The initial biochemical events following TCR stimulation, such as induction of the second messengers IP3 and DAG, have been described to be either severely compromised [38] or unaffected by aging [39]. These contrasting results may reflect the use of different experimental procedures. Both the GPTase activity and the level of G proteins were found to change in lymphocytes from old individuals, the most significant alterations being found in the amounts of Gi and Gq subtypes [40].

Table 2

Effect of aging on signal transduction in anti-CD3-activated T cells

Membrane		**Cytoplasm**		**Nucleus**	
PLC-γ1 expression	↓	SHC phosphorylation	↓	NF-AT	↓
Phosphorylation	↓	p56^{lck} phosphorylation	↓	AP-1	↓
Intrinsic enzymatic activity	=	p59^{fyn} phosphorylation	↓	NFkB	↓
PIP_2 expression	=	ZAP-70 expression	=	IkB-α	↑
IP_3 production	↓ /=	phosphorylation	↓	c-fos	=
DAG production		Grb-2 phosphorylation	↓	c-jun	↓
Ca^{++} mobilization	↓	Raf-1 expression	↑	c-myc	↓
G proteins	↓	kinase activity	↓	Oct-1	=
		MAPK/ERK kinase activity	↓		
		MAP phosphatase activity	↑		
		PKCα translocation	↓		
		PKCβ translocation	=		
		PKCγ translocation	↓		
		PKCζ translocation	↓		

Studies on PKC isoforms (α, β, γ, ζ) revealed different profiles in lymphocytes from young and old individuals [40]. Only the PKCβ, but not the other isoforms, is able to translocate into the nucleus of activated lymphocytes from elderly subjects, whereas all the isoforms can translocate into the nucleus of activated lymphocytes from adult controls.

We have studied the effects of aging on the activation of the cytoplasmatic tyrosine protein kinase p56^{lck} in PBL from adult and elderly subjects. Results [41] show that the amount and phosphorylation of p56^{lck} is reduced in PBL from elderly as compared to adult subjects, suggesting that alterations in p56^{lck} may contribute to the age-associated loss of some T cell function, such as proliferation and IL-2 production, which are found to be decreased in PBL from old individuals. However, p56^{lck} seems irrelevant to the production of IFN-γ and IL-4 which were both found to be increased in the PBL from old subjects, as expected from the relative expansion of memory *versus* naive T cell subpopulations in aging.

Signal trasduction pathways mediated by the family of mitogen-activated protein kinases (MAPK) and the multifunctional MEK family, which is composed of MAPK/extracellular regulated kinases (ERK), have been found to be reduced in aging [42] in terms of both levels and duration of active MAPK. Since no age-related differences were found in the expression of p42^{mapk}/ERK2, p44^{mapk}/ERK1 or MEK, the impairment appears in the upstream inducers of MEK/MAPK activation. An increased expression of MAP phosphatase, which counteracts kinase activity, has also been reported to occur in aging [43].

Reduced activation of several transcriptional factors involved in the regulation of gene transcription has been found in aging. Among these factors, AP-1 and NF-AT are decreased in T cells from old individuals [42, 44]. This age-related decline in the induction of DNA binding activity of the transcription factors AP-1 and NF-AT has also been described in old rats and attributed to changes in the expression of $p21^{ras}$ kinase signaling pathway [45]. Also the nuclear NF-kB is decreased in aging and may be attributed to a higher activity of the IkB-α inhibitor in aging [46]. Unlike c-fos, c-jun [47] and c-myc [44] are decreased in old individuals, whereas OCT-1 seems to be unaffected by aging [46, 48].

The decreased T cell immunity is also associated with shifts in T cell subsets and cytokine secretion profiles (Table 3).

Table 3
Cytokine production by naive and memory T cells in aging mice

T cells	Young			Old		
	IL-2	IFN-γ	IL-4	IL-2	IFN-γ	IL-4
Naive*	++++	+	++	+	++	++++
Memory**	++	++	++++	++	++++	++

*: $CD44^{low}$, $CD45RB^{high}$, $Mel\text{-}14^{high}$, $3G11^{high}$
**: $CD44^{high}$, $CD45RB^{low}$, $Mel\text{-}14^{low}$, $3G11^{low}$

Changes in the splenic T cell population have been shown to be a consequence of thymus involution [49] and to consist of a gradual decline in cell number with an increase of the CD4/CD8 cell ratio, due to a relative decrease in the CD8+ cell number [50]. Although the percent of splenic CD4+ cell does not change greatly with age, the composition of this cell subpopulation is quite different in young and old mice. The peripheral pool of CD4+ naive T cells ($CD44^{low}$ $CD45RB^{high}$ $MEL\text{-}14^{high}$ $3G11^{high}$), which has been shown to be predominant in young mice, decreases with age while that of memory T cells ($CD44^{high}$ $CD45^{low}$ MEL-14 ^{low} $3G11^{low}$) increases [51, 52]. Similar changes in naive and memory T cell subpopulations have also been found to occur in the peripheral pool of CD8+ cells of aging mice [53]. Studies on the role of the thymus in age-related changes of the naive and memory T cell pools [54] have indicated that the young thymus has a greater propensity to provide naive T cells as compared to the old thymus that, instead, favors the differentiation and maintenance of memory T cells rather than naive T cells.

In humans, it is difficult to assess the contribution of thymic involution to changes in T cell functions. However, there is evidence suggesting that even in very old individuals sufficient thymic function may be retained to allow naive T cell differentiation [55].

Analysis of PBL, as performed in aging humans [56, 57], has shown that the absolute numbers of CD4+ and CD8+ T cells, and B cells decrease, while those of NK cells increase with age, from 20 to 100 years. As observed in the mouse, the percent of naive T cells decreases while that of memory T cells increases with age in both CD4+ and CD8+ cell populations (Fig. 1).

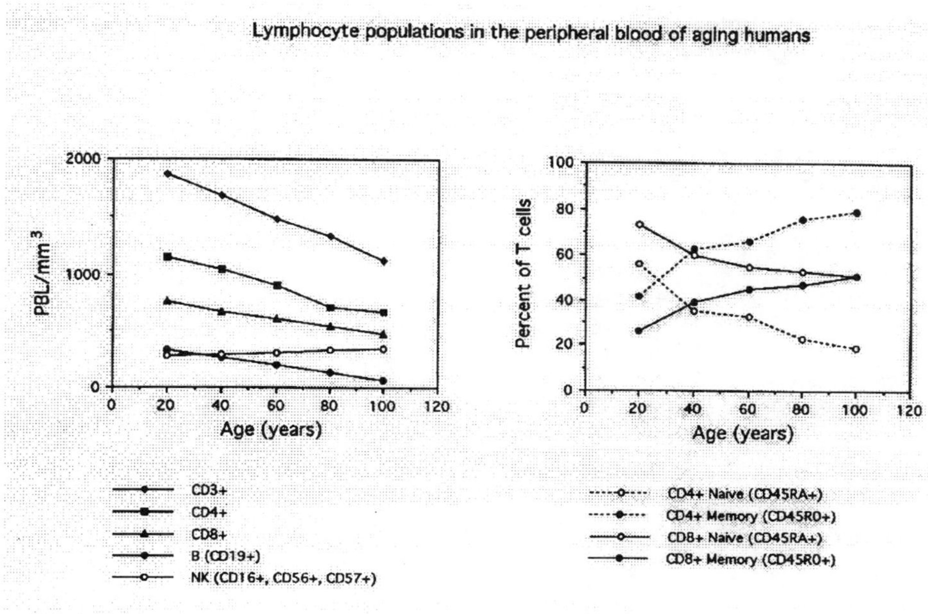

Fig. 1

Recently, we have investigated the ability of naive and memory T cell populations from subjects of different ages to be activated *in vitro* by cross-linking of CD3, alone or in combination with the recombinant human cytokines IL-1β, IL-2, IL-3, IL-4, IL-12, or by the cytokines alone. Results in Table 4 show that in young (aged 25-35 years) subjects the mitotic response elicited by memory T cells is greater than that elicited by naive T cells. Moreover, the response of naive and memory T cells may be enhanced by the addition of IL-2 and IL-12. The cytokines are devoid of mitogenic activities when used alone. Results in Table 5 demonstrate that also in old (aged 67-93 years) subjects the mitotic response elicited in memory T cells is greater than that elicited in naive T cells and can be enhanced by addition of IL-2. This effect of IL-2 is more pronounced for naive T cells.

Table 4
Mitotic responses of naive (CD45RA+) and memory (CD45RO+) T cells purified from the peripheral blood of young donors.

Subject	Cell proliferation induced by	Cells in culture CD45RA+	CD45RO+
1	-	95 ± 6	113 ± 2
	anti-CD3	2889 ± 272	4797 ± 231
	anti-CD3/IL-1	3228 ± 101	5041 ± 148
	anti-CD3/IL-2	3439 ± 44	5652 ± 344
	anti-CD3/IL-4	2848 ± 134	4286 ± 117
	anti-CD3/IL-12	3441 ± 154	5832 ± 508
	IL-1	153 ± 20	145 ± 18
	IL-2	111 ± 6	121 ± 1
	IL-4	108 ± 13	133 ± 1
	IL-12	123 ± 21	199 ± 1
2	-	89 ± 6	100 ± 3
	anti-CD3	2776 ± 180	4922 ± 192
	anti-CD3/IL-1	3234 ± 114	5111 ± 182
	anti-CD3/IL-2	3117 ± 276	5128 ± 99
	anti-CD3/IL-4	2843 ± 198	4465 ± 321
	anti-CD3/IL-12	3621 ± 275	5799 ± 290
3	-	93 ± 9	99 ± 10
	anti-CD3	2991 ± 186	5013 ± 166
	anti-CD3/IL-1	3457 ± 220	5187 ± 308
	anti-CD3/IL-2	3927 ± 197	5222 ± 231
	anti-CD3/IL-4	2933 ± 224	4977 ± 128
	anti-CD3/IL-12	4213 ± 385	5992 ± 130
4	-	101 ± 7	98 ± 8
	anti-CD3	3077 ± 233	4923 ± 118
	anti-CD3/IL-1	4032 ± 127	5418 ± 239
	anti-CD3/IL-2	4437 ± 102	6032 ± 166
	anti-CD3/IL-4	2718 ± 223	4532 ± 311
	anti-CD3/IL-12	4677 ± 274	6320 ± 219

Results are expressed as cpm and are means from triplicate cultures ± S.E.
All cytokines were used at the concentration of 60 U/ml.

The results in Table 4 and 5 indicate that it is possible to activate naive and memory T cells from both young and old subjects in vitro by cross-linking of CD3. The addition of recombinant cytokines is an effective co-stimulus for naive T cells from old subjects and, to a lesser extent, for naive and memory T cells from young subjects. These results underscore the potential use of cytokines as adjuvants in vaccination.

Table 5
Mitotic responses of naive (CD45RA+) and memory (CD45RO+) T cells purified from the peripheral blood of elderly donors.

Subject	Cell proliferation induced by	Cells in culture CD45RA+	CD45RO+
1	-	72 ± 2	103 ± 3
	anti-CD3	1884 ± 44	3256 ± 129
	anti-CD3/IL-2	2380 ± 253	3637 ± 225
2	-	81 ± 4	102 ± 5
	anti-CD3	1789 ± 92	3679 ± 171
	anti-CD3/IL-2	2662 ± 124	4021 ± 194
3	-	76 ± 5	79 ± 9
	anti-CD3	1668 ± 134	3412 ± 568
	anti-CD3/IL-2	2481 ± 97	4029 ± 143
4	-	69 ± 6	81 ± 6
	anti-CD3	1854 ± 132	3536 ± 103
	anti-CD3/IL-2	2570 ± 143	4013 ± 166

Results are expressed as cpm and are means from triplicate cultures ± S.E.
IL-2 was used at the concentration of 60 U/ml.

The age-related alteration of the peripheral CD4+ T helper cell subsets in terms of cell surface phenotype and cytokine production, as they emerge from the aging thymus, may produce suitable conditions for T cell-mediated dysregulation of antibody responses. Hence, an inbalance within the CD4+ T cell population may reduce B cell proliferation and mutation rate during the antibody response, leading to the production of low affinity antibodies with increased cross-reactivity to self antigens [58-60]. Although in some cases autoantibodies are of the IgM isotype, the response to many, if not all, autoantigens requires T cell help [61]. The appearance of autoreactive T cells in the periphery [62, 63] is often concomitant with the infiltration of organs by CD4+ T cells [64] although evidence of the organ-specific reactivity of these cells is lacking. It is likely that autoimmunity is induced and prevented by the interplay of autoreactive and regulatory CD4+ T cell subsets [65].

The antibody response to exogenous antigens is decreased in aging, but it is uncertain to what extent this decline reflects changes in the performance of T cells needed to promote B cell activation and differentiation [66], or intrinsic changes in B cell function [67]. A negative effect of age on signal transduction pathways involving Ca^{++}-dependent PKC has been demonstrated in murine B cells [68]. Moreover, studies on B cell hybridomas [69] and single B cells [70] have indicated that individual cells from aging mice are increasingly likely to produce antibodies with low affinity and cross-reactive specificity for foreign and self antigens. Limited data [71] suggest that aging may lead to major changes in the molecular processes by which antibody genes are assembled and then selected. Impairment of B cell generation in bone marrow of old mice, as shown at the level of pro- and pre-B cells [72], may induce qualitative as well as quantitative alterations affecting tolerance and responsiveness of the mature B cell population.

The ability of accessory cells to support T and B cell activation seems unaffected by aging [17]. However, the observed defects in the ability of follicular dendritic cells to process and present immune complexes may contribute to the decline of germinal center formation in old mice [58, 73]. Furthermore, the defects in the transport of antigens into lymph node germinal centers by migrating dendritic cells may also contribute to decrease of humoral and cell-mediated immunity [74].

Studies on natural killer (NK) cell function in old mice have shown a profound loss of NK cell function when spleen and lymph node cells were assayed, suggesting that a loss of NK cell activity contributes to increasing sensitivity to neoplastic and viral diseases [75, 76]. In humans, however, the number of NK cells in peripheral blood has been shown to increase with aging, while NK activity is decreased in the elderly [77]. This loss of NK activity has been attributed to the impairment in the phosphoinositide signaling pathway, in particular to reduced IP3 levels, whereas the intracellular content of perforin seems to be unaffected by aging [78].

5. Cytokine production and expression of cytokine receptors in aging.

Accessory cell-derived cytokines.

Studies on monocyte/macrophage-derived cytokines have yielded controversial results, as the aging effects on these cell populations are extremely dependent upon variations in stimuli, culture conditions and cytokines produced. IL-1 production by macrophages from old mice was found to be unchanged [17] or decreased [79] as compared to young controls. Moreover, it has recently been demonstrated that macrophages from old mice constitutively produce higher levels of both p35 and p40 IL-12 mRNA, as compared to young mice [80], which may account, at least in part, for altered production of T cell-derived cytokines in aging. The spontaneous release of IL-8 by monocytes is reduced in aging but the LPS-induced release is higher in old as compared to young individuals [81]. Moreover, the monocyte- and lymphocyte-derived TNF-α seems to be increased in aging [82]. TNFR p55 and p75 were found to be unaffected by aging in murine CD8+ spleen cells [83].

T cell-derived cytokines.

T cell proliferation declines with aging in both mice [17, 84-87], and humans [88, 89]. Cell cycle analysis of PHA-stimulated cells from old individuals indicates a decreased frequency of cells entering the S phase. The age-related impairment in the cell cycle progression correlates with decreased expression not only of c-myc (G0/G1 progression marker) and c-myb (G1/S progression marker), but also of c-jun, IL-2 production and IL-2R expression [48, 90, 91].

Alteration in T cell proliferation with aging leads to dysregulation but not necessarily to reduction of cytokine production. Most of the results obtained in both humans and rodents show reduced IL-2 production and increased IL-4 production with aging [88, 92-99]. However, many controversial results concerning reduced or unchanged IL-4 release in aging have also been reported and primarily reflect differences in stimuli and methods of determination [92, 99, 100]. Young naive T cells produce mainly IL-2 whereas young memory T cells mainly IL-4. At variance, in old mice memory T cells produce twice as much IL-2 than naive T cells, while the overall level of IL-2 is significantly lower than that in young mice. Moreover, in old mice naive T cells produce twice as much IL-4 than memory T cells, while the overall level of IL-4 is at least the same as that in young mice.

The number and/or affinity of IL-2R expression on the surface of activated lymphocytes declines with aging in both mice and humans [101, 102]. The release of the soluble form of the IL-2R (sIL-2R) in culture supernatants of activated human lymphocytes has been reported to decline [92, 103] or to increase [104] with aging. IL-4R mRNA has been described to be similarly expressed in murine CD8+ splenocytes from young and old mice [83]. IFN-γ has been described to increase during aging [54, 71, 99, 105], although it was found to be decreased [92, 106] or unchanged [107] in some studies. The mRNA level for IFN-γR is unaffected by aging in murine CD8+ splenocytes [83]. The release of hematopoietic cytokines such as IL-3 [108] and GM-CFS [67] seems severely affected by aging. However, IL-3 has also been reported to increase in aging [95]. IL-5 increases with aging [95] while IL-6 has been reported to be unaffected [95] or increased [67] by aging. Also the anti-inflammatory cytokine IL-10 increases in the serum of old, as compared to young, individuals [70], suggesting that the higher resistance to the septic shock in aging may be due, at least in part, to increased levels of this protective cytokine.

6. Concluding remarks

During senescence, alterations of the immune system affect both antibody and cell-mediated responses. Within the T cell population, aging leads to the replacement of virgin cells by memory cells, and to the accumulation of cells with signal transduction defects. Age-related changes in T cell subpopulations and in the cytokine profile may produce suitable conditions for T cell-mediated dysregulation of antibody responses characterized by the production of low affinity and self-reactive antibodies. Also, B cells and NK cells display profound alterations during the aging process.

References

[1] R.A. Miller, The Biology of Aging and Longevity. In: R. W. Hazzard (ed.) Principles of geriatric medicine and gerontology, 3rd edition. Mc Graw-Hill, Inc., New York, 1994, pp.3-18.

[2] L. Hayflick, Prospects for Human Life Extension by Genetic Manipulation. In: D. Danon, NW Shock, M. Marois (eds), Aging: a challenge to science and society. Vol. 1 Biology. Oxford Univ. Press, New York, 1981, pp. 162-179.

[3] L.E. Orgel, The Maintenance of the Accuracy of Protein Synthesis and its Relevance to Aging, *Proc Natl Acad Sci USA* **49** (1963) 517-520.

[4] S.M. Jazwinski, Longevity, Genes and Aging, *Science* **273** (1996) 54-59.

[5] R.A. Miller, The Aging Immune System: Primer and Prospectus. *Science* **273** (1996) 70-74.

[6] G.S. Smith, R.L. Walford, Influence of the Main Histocompatibility Complex on Aging Mice, *Nature* **270** (1977) 727-729.

[7] R.L. Walford, R.H. Weindruch, S.R.S. Gottesman, C.F. Tam. The Immunopathology of Aging, *Annu Rev Gerontol Geriat* **2** (1981) 3-14.

[8] D. Harman, The Aging Process, *Proc Natl Acad Sci USA* **78** (1981) 7124-7128.

[9] C.F. Tam, R.L. Walford, Cyclic Nucleotide Levels in Resting and Mitogen-Stimulated Cell Suspensions from Young and Old Mice, *Mech Ageing Dev,* **7** (1978) 309-320.

[10] R.L. Walford, K. Bergmann, Influences of Genes Associated with the Main Histocompatibility Complex on Deoxyribonucleic Acid Excision Repair Capacity and Bleomycin Sensitivity in Mouse Lymphocytes, *Tissue Antigens* **14** (1979) 336-342.

[11] R.W. Hart, R.B. Setlow, Correlation between Deoxyribonucleic Acid Excision Repair and Lifespan in a Number of Mammalian Species, *Proc Natl Acad Sci USA*, **71** (1974) 2169-2173.

[12] S.P. Jackson, The Recognition of DNA Damage, *Current Opinion in Genetics and Development* **6** (1996) 19-25.

[13] DNA repair, a special issue. *Trends Biochem Sci* .**237** (1995).

[14] D. Frasca, P. Barattini, C. Goso, S. Pucci, G. Rizzo, C. Bartoloni, M. Costanzo, A. Errani, L. Guidi, L. Antico, A. Tricerri, G. Doria, Cell Proliferation and Ku Protein Expression in Ageing Humans, *Mech Ageing Dev* **93** (1998) 157-169..

[15] D. Frasca, P. Barattini, D. Tirindelli, L. Guidi, C. Bartoloni, A. R. Errani, M. Costanzo, A. Tricerri, L. Pierelli, G. Doria, Effect of age on DNA binding of the ku protein in irradiated human peripheral blood lymphocytes (submitted to Exp. Gerontology)

[16] R.L. Walford, Immunological Theory of Aging: Current Status, *Fed. Proc* **33** (1974) 2020-2027.

[17] G. Doria, L. Adorini, D. Frasca, Immunoregulation of Antibody Responses in Aging Mice. In: E.A. Goidl (ed.), Aging and the Immune Response. Cellular and Humoral Aspects. Marcel Dekker, Inc, New York, 1987, pp. 143-176.

[18] G. Doria, C. Mancini, M. Utsuyama, D. Frasca, K. Hirokawa, Aging of the Recipients but not of the Bone Marrow Donors Enhances Autoimmunity in Syngeneic Radiation Chimeras, *Mech Ageing Dev* **95** (1997) 131-142.

[19] M.E. Weskler, Immunesenescense, *Ann. Neurol* **35** (1994) 35-37.

[20] T. Makinodan, W.H. Adler, Effects of Aging on the Differentiation and Proliferation Potentials of Cells of the Immune System, *Fed Proc* **34** (1975) 153-158.

[21] T. Makinodan, J.W. Albright, P.I. Good, C.P. Peter, M.L. Heidrick, Reduced Humoral Immune Reactivity in Long-Lived Old Mice: an Approach to Elucidating its Mechanisms, *Immunology* **31** (1976) 903-911

[22] R.E. Callard, Aging of the Immune System. In: M.M.B. Kay, T. Makinodan (eds.). Handbook of Immunology in Aging. CRC Press, Boca Raton, FL, 1981, pp. 103-113.

[23] M.M.B. Kay, T. Makinodan, The Ageing Immune System. In: A. Viidik (ed.), Lectures on Gerontology. Vol. I: On Biology of Ageing. Part A, Acad Press, Orlando, FL, 1982, pp. 143-171.

[24] D.E. Harrison, Long-Term Erythropoietic Repopulating Ability of Old, Young and Fetal Stem Cells, *J Exp Med* **157** (1983) 1496-1504.

[25] R. Eren, D. Zharhary, L. Abel, A. Globerson, Age-Related Changes in the Capacity of Bone Marrow Cells to Differentiate in Thymic Organ Cultures, *Cell Immunol* **112** (1988) 449-455.

[26] A. Keating, The Hematopoietic Stem Cell in Elderly Patients with Leukemia, *Leukemia* **10** (1996) S30-S32.

[27] M.L. Thoman, W.O. Weigle, The Cellular and Subcellular Bases of Immunosenescence, *Adv Immunol* **46** (1989) 221-261.

[28] R.A. Miller, Age-Associated Decline in Precorsor Fequency for Different T Cell-Mediated Reactions, with Preservation of Helper and Cytotoxic Effect per Precursor Cell, *J Immunol* **132** (1984) 63-68.

[29] R.A. Miller, Immunodeficiency of Aging: Restorative Effects of Phorbol Ester Combined with Calcium Ionophore, *J Immunol* **137** (1986) 805-808.

[30] M.L. Thoman, W.O. Weigle, Partial Restoration of ConA-Induced Proliferation, IL-2 Receptor Expression, and IL-2 Synthesis in Aged Murine Lymphocytes by Phorbol Myristate Acetate and Ionomycin, *Cell Immunol* **114** (1988) 1-11.

[31] R.A. Miller, B. Jacobson, G. Weil, E.R. Simons, Diminished Calcium Influx in Lectin-Stimulated T Cells from Old Mice, *J Cell Physiol* **132** (1987) 337-342.

[32] J.J. Proust, C.R. Filburn, S.A. Harrison, M.A. Bucholz, A.A. Nordin, Age-Related Defect in Signal Transduction During Lectin Activation of Murine T Lymphocytes, *J Immunol* **139** (1987) 1472-1478.

[33] B. Philosophe, R.A. Miller, Diminished Calcium Signal Generation in Subsets of T Lymphocytes that Predominate in Old Mice, *J Gerontol Biol Sci* **45** (1990) B87-B89.

[34] B. Philosophe, R.A. Miller, Calcium Signals in Murine T Lymphocytes: Preservation of Responses to PHA and to an Anti-ly-6 Antibody, *Aging: Immunol Infect Dis* **2** (1991) 11-18.

[35] J. Shi, R.A. Miller, Differential Tyrosine-Specific Protein Phosphorylation in Mouse T Lymphocytes Subsets. Effect of Age, *J Immunol* **151** (1993) 730-739.

[36] G.G. Garcia, R.A. Miller, Differential Tyrosine Phosphorylation of Zeta Chain Dimers in Mouse CD4 T Lymphocytes: Effect of Age, *Cell Immunol* **175** (1997) 51-57.

[37] H.R. Patel, R.A. Miller, Age-Associated Changes in Mitogen-Induced Protein Phosphorylation in Murine T Lymphocytes, *Eur J Immunol* **22** (1992) 253-260.

[38] R.A. Miller, Aging and Immune Function, *Int Rev Cytol* **124** (1991) 187-216.

[39] M. Utsuyama, Z. Varga,K. Fukami,Y. Homma, T. Takenawa, K. Hirokawa, Influence of Age on the Signal Transduction of T Cells in Mice, *Int Immunol* **5** (1993) 1177-1182.

[40] T. Fulop, Signal Transduction Changes in Granulocytes and Lymphocytes with Ageing, *Immunol Letters* **40** (1994) 259-268.

[41] L. Guidi, L. Antico, C. Bartoloni, M. Costanzo, A. Errani, A. Tricerri, M. Vangeli, G. Doria, L. Gatta, C. Goso, L. Mancino, D. Frasca, Changes in the Amount and Level of Phosphorylation of $p56^{lck}$ in PBL from Aging Humans, *Mech Ageing Dev* **102** (1998) 177-186.

[42] R.L. Whisler, Y.G. Newhouse, S.E. Bagenstose, Age-Related Reductions in the Activation of Mitogen-Activated Protein Kinases $p44^{mapk}$/ERK1 and $p42^{mapk}$/ERK2 in Human T Cells Stimulated via Ligation of the T Cell Receptor Complex, *Cell Immunol* **168** (1996) 201-210.

[43] Y.S. Liu, K.Z. Guyton, M. Gorospe, Age-Related Decline in Mitogen-Activated Protein Kinase Activity in Epidermal Growth Factor-Stimulated Rat Hepatocytes, *J Biol Chem* **271** (1996) 3604-3607.

[44] R.L. Whisler, L. Beiqing, L.C. Wu, M. Chen, Reduced Activation of Transcriptional Factor AP-1 Among Peripheral Blood T Cells From Elderly Humans after PHA Stimulation: Restorative Effect of Phorbol Diesters, *Cell Immunol* **152** (1993) 96-109.

[45] M.A. Palhavani, M.D. Harris, A. Richardson, The Age-Related Decline in the Induction of DNA Dinding Activity of the Transcription Factors AP-1 and NFAT is Correlated to Changes in the Expression of $p21^{ras}$/MAP Kinase Signalling Tathway. In: First International Conference on Immunology and Aging. Bethesda MD, 1996, pp. 1-13.

[46] G.U. Trebilcock, U. Ponnappan, Nuclear factors-kB induction in CD45R0+ and CD45RA+ T cell subsets, *Mech Ageing Dev* **102** (1998) 149-163.

[47] L.J. Song, J.M. Stephens, S. Kittur, Expression of c-fos, c-jun and jun-b in PBL from Young and Elderly Adults, *Mech Ageing Dev* **65** (1992) 149-156.

[48] G.U. Trebilcock, U. Ponnappan, Evidence for Lowered Induction of Nuclear Factor Kappa B in Activated Human T Lymphocytes During Aging, *Gerontology* **42** (1996) 137-146.

[49] M. Utsuyama, M. Kasai, C. Kurashima, K. Hirokawa, Age Influence on the Thymic Capacity to Promote Differentiation of T Cells: Induction of Different Composition of T Cell Subsets by Aging Thymus, *Mech Ageing Dev* **58** (1991) 267-277.

[50] M. Utsuyama, K. Hirokawa, Age-Related Changes of Splenic T Cells in Mice. A Flow Cytometric Analysis, *Mech Ageing Dev* **40** (1987) 89-102.

[51] D.N. Ernst, M.V. Hobbs, B.E. Torbett, A.L. Glasebrook, M.A. Rehse, K. Bottomly, K. Hayakawa, R.R. Hardy, W.O. Weigle, Differences in the Expression Profiles of CD45RB, Pgp-1 and 3G11 Membrane Antigens and in the Patterns of Lymphokine Secretion by Splenic CD4+ T Cells from Young and Aged Mice, *J Immunol* **145** (1990) 1295-1302.

[52] D.N. Ernst, M.V. Hobbs, B.E. Torbett, A.L. Glasebrook, M.A. Rehse, D.N. McQuitty, K. Bottomly, W.O. Weigle, Differences in the Subset Composition of CD4+ T Cell Populations from Young and Old Mice, *Aging: Immunol Infect Dis* **2** (1990) 105-109.

[53] D.N. Ernst, W.O. Weigle, D.J. Noonan, D.N. McQuitty, M.V. Hobbs, The Age-Associated Increase in IFN-γ Synthesis by Mouse CD8+ T Cells Correlates with Shifts in the Frequencies of Cell Subsets Defined by Membrane CD44, CD45RB, 3G11 and Mel-14 Expression, *J Immunol* **151** (1993) 575-587.

[54] C. Kurashima, M. Utsuyama, M. Kasai, S.A. Ishyima, A. Konno, K. Hirokawa, The Role of Thymus in the Aging of Th Cell Subpopulations and Age-Associated Alterations of Cytokine Production by these Cells. *Int Immunol* **7** (1995) 97-104.

[55] G. Steinmann, M. Hartwig. Immunology of Centenarians, *Immunol Today* **16** (1995) 549-552.

[56] P. Sansoni, A. Cossarizza, V. Brianti, F. Fagnoni, G. Snelli, D. Monti, A. Marcato, G. Passeri, C. Ortolani, E. Forti, U. Fagiolo, M. Passeri, C. Franceschi. Lymphocyte Subsets and Natural Killer Cell Activity in Healthy Old People and Centenarians. *Blood* **80** (1993) 2767-2773.

[57] A. Cossarizza, C. Ortolani, R. Paganelli, D. Barbieri, D. Monti, U. Fagiolo, G. Castellani, F. Bersani, P. Sansoni, M. Londei, C. Franceschi, CD45 Isoforms Expression on CD4+ and CD8+ T Cells throughout Life from Newborns to Centenarians: Implications for T Cell Memory, *Mech Ageing Dev* **86** (1996) 173-195.

[58] C. Miller, G. Kelsoe, S. Han, Lack of B7-2 Expression in the Germinal Centers of Aged Mice, *Aging: Immunol Infect Dis* **5** (1994) 249-257.

[59] C. Miller, G. Kelsoe, IgVH Hypermutation is Absent in the Germinal Centers of Aged Mice, *J Immunol* **155** (1995) 3377-3384.

[60] X. Yang, J. Streda, J. Cerny, Relative Contribution of T and B Cells to Hypermutation and Selection of the Antibody Repertoire in Germinal Centers of Aged Mice, *J Exp Med* **183** (1996) 959-970.

[61] M.E. Weksler, The Nature and Significance of Age-Associated Autoimmunity. In: C.A. Bona, K. Siminovitch, M. Zanetti, A.N. Theofilopoulos (eds.), Molecular Pathology of Autoimmunity Diseases. Hardwood Acad Publ, New York, 1993, 765-775.

[62] D. Naor, B. Bonavida, R.L. Walford, Autoimmunity and Aging: the Age-Related Response of Mice of a Long-Lived Strain to Trinitrophenylated Syngeneic Mouse Red Blood Cells, *J Immunol* **117** (1976) 2204-2208.

[63] J. Charreire, J.F. Bach, Binding of Autologous Erythrocytes to Immature T Cells, *Proc Natl Acad Sci USA* **72** (1975) 3201-3205.

[64] Y. Hayashi, M. Utsuyama, C. Kurashima, K. Hirokawa, Spontaneous Development of Organ-Specific Autoimmune Lesions in Aged C57BL/6 Mice, *Clin Exp Immunol* **78** (1989) 120-126.
[65] D. Fowell, A.J. McNight, F. Powrie, R. Dyke, D. Mason, Subsets of CD4+ T Cells and their Roles in the Induction and Prevention of Autoimmunity, *Immunol Rev* **123** (1991) 37-64.
[66] S.P. Li, S. Verma, R.A. Miller, Age-Related Defects in T Cell Expression of CD40 Ligand and Induction of in Vitro B Cell Activation, *Aging: Immunol Infect Dis* **6** (1995) 79-93.
[67] N.R. Klinman, The Basis for Decreased B Cell Responsiveness with Aging: the Legacy and the Challenge, *Aging: Immunol Infec Dis* **5** (1994) 203-210.
[68] H. Kawanishi, K. Joseph., Effects of Phorbol Myristate and Ionomycin on in Vitro Growth of Aged Peyer's Patch T and B Cells, *Mech Ageing Dev,* **65** (1992) 289-300.
[69] S.J.M. McElvoy, E.A. Goidl, Studies on Immunological Maturation. II. The Absence of High-Affinity Antibody Producing Cells Early in the Immune Response is Only Apparent, *Aging Immunol Infect Dis* **1** (1988) 47-54.
[70] N.R. Klinman, Similarties in B Cell Repertoire Development Between Autoimmune and Aging Normal Mice, *J Immunol* **148** (1992) 1353-1358.
[71] L.A. Bangs, I.E. Sanz, J.M. Teale, Comparison of D, JH, and Junctional Diversity in the Fetal, Adult, and Aged B Cell Repertoires, *J Immunol* **146** (1991) 1996-2004.
[72] D. Zharhary, Age-Related Changes in the Capability of the Bone Marrow to Generate B Cells, *J Immunol* **141** (1988) 1863-1869.
[73] G.F. Burton, M.H. Kosco, A.K. Szakal, J.C. Tew, Iccosomes and the Secondary Antibody Response, *Immunology* **73** (1991) 271-276.
[74] K.L. Holmes, C.T. Schnizlein, E.H. Perkins, J.C. Tew, The Effect of Age on Antigen Retention in Lymphoid Follicles and in Collagenous Tissue of Mice, *Mech Ageing Dev* **25** (1984) 243-255.
[75] R. Weindruch, B.H. Devens, H.V. Raff, R.L. Walford, Influence of DietaryRestriction and Aging on Nautral Killer Cell Activity in Mice, *J Immunol* **130** (1983) 993-996.
[76] J.W. Albright, J.F. Albright, Age-Associated Impairment of Murine Natural Killer Activity, *Proc Natl Acad Sci USA* **80** (1983) 6371-6375.
[77] A. Facchini, E. Mariani, A.R. Mariani, S. Papa, M. Vitale, F.A. Manzoli, Increased Number of Circulating Leu 11+ (CD16) Large Granular Lymphocytes and Decreased NK Activity During Human Ageing, *Clin exp Immunol* **68** (1987) 340-347.
[78] A. Facchini, A.R. Mariani, A. Tarozzi, M. Tadolini, A. Meneghetti, E. Podack, E. Mariani, Signal Transduction and Perforin Release After NK Cell Activation During Ageing, In*: 9th International Congress of Immunology*, S. Francisco (1995) 206.
[79] T. Inamizu, M.-P. Chang, T. Makinodan, Influence of Age on the Production and Regulation of IL-1 in Mice, *Immunology* **55** (1985) 447-455.
[80] N.F.L. Spencer, R.A. Daynes, IL-12 Directly Stimulates Expression of IL-10 by CD5+ B Cells and IL-6 by Both CD5+ and CD5- B Cells: Possible Involvement in Age-Associated Cytokine Disregulation, *Int Immunol* (1997) in press.
[81] J.A. Clark, T.C. Peterson, Cytokine Production and Aging. Overproduction of IL-8 in Elderly Males in Response to LPS *Mech Ageing Dev* **77** (1994) 127-139.
[82] D. Han, T. Hosokawa, A. Aoike, K. Kawai, Age-Related Enhancement of TNF Production in Mice, *Mech Ageing Dev* **84** (1995) 39-54.
[83] D.N. Ernst, D.W. Sehv, W.O. Weigle, Aging, Cytokine and Cytokine Receptor Expression by Mouse CD8+ Cells, In*: 9th International Congress of Immunology*, S. Francisco (1995) 196.
[84] R.E. Callard, Immune Function in Aged Mice, *Eur J Immunol* **8** (1978) 697-705.
[85] R.L. Krogsrud, E.H. Perkins, Age-Related Changes in T Cell Functions, *J Immunol* **118** (1977) 1607-1611.
[86] D. Frasca, L. Adorini, S. Landolfo, G. Doria, Enhancing Effect of IFN-γ on Helper T Cell Activity and IL-2 Production, *J Immunol* **134** (1985) 3907-3911.
[87] C. Goso, D. Frasca, G. Doria, Effect of Synthetic Thymic Humoral Factor (THF-γ2) on T Cell Activities in Immunodeficient Ageing Mice, *Clin exp Immunol* **87** (1992) 346-351.
[88] W. Barcellini, M.O. Borghi, C. Sguotti, R. Palmieri, D. Frasca, P.L. Meroni, G. Doria, C. Zanussi, Heterogeneity of Immune Responsiveness in Healthy Elderly Subjects, *Clin Immunol Immunopathol* **47** (1988) 142-151.
[89] C. Bartoloni, L. Guidi, D. Frasca, L. Antico, R. Pili, F Cursi, A. Di Giovanni, C. Rumi, E. Menini, P.U. Carbonin, G. Doria, G. Gambassi, Immune Parameters in a Population of Institutionalized Elderly Subjects: Influence of Depressive Disorders and Endocrinological Correlations, *Mech Ageing Dev* **60** (1991) 1-12.
[90] D.A. Gamble, R. Schwab, M.E. Weksler, P. Szabo, Decreased Steady State c-myc mRNA in Activated T Cell Cultures from Old Humans is Caused by a Smaller Proportion of T Cells that Transcribe the c-myc Gene, *J Immunol* **144** (1990) 3569-3573.

[91] C. Pieri, R. Recchioni, F. Moroni, F Marcheselli, G. Lipponi, Phytohemagglutinin Induced Changes of Membrane Lipid Packing, c-myc and c-myb Encoded Protein Expression in Human Lymphocytes During Aging, *Mech Ageing Dev* **64** (1992) 177-187.

[92] R.A. Daynes, B.A. Araneo, Prevention and Reversal of Some Age-Associated Changes in Immunologic Responses by Supplemental Dehydroepiandrosterone Sulfate Therapy. Aging, *Immuno Infect Dis* **3** (1992) 135-154.

[93] M.P. Chang, T. Makinodan, W.J. Peterson, B.L.Strehler, Role of T Cells and Adherent Cells in Age-Related Decline in Murine Interleukin-2 Production, *J Immunol* **129** (1982) 2426-2430.

[94] M.L. Thoman, W.O. Weigle. Lymphokines and Aging: Interleukin-2 Production and Activity in Aged Animals, *J Immunol* **127** (1991) 2102-2106.

[95] M.V. Hobbs, W.O. Weigle, D.J. Noonan, B.E. Torbett, R.J. McEvilly, R.J. Koch, G.J. Cardenas, D.N. Ernst, Patterns of Cytokine Gene Expression by CD4+ T Cells from Young and Old Mice, *J Immunol* **150** (1993) 3602-3614.

[96] L. Nagelkerken, A. Hertogh-Huijbregts, R. Dobber, A. Drager, Age-Related Changes in Lymphokine Production Related to a Decreased Number of $CD45RB^{hi}$ CD4+ T Cells, *Eur J Immunol*, **21** (1991) 273-281.

[97] M. Kubo, B. Cinader, Polymorphism of Age-Related Changes in Interleukin (IL) Production: Differential Changes of T Helper Subpopulations Synthesizing IL-2, IL-3 and IL-4, *Eur J Immunol* **20** (1990) 1289-1296.

[98] I. Kirman, K.S. Zhao, I. Tschepen, P. Szabo, G. Richter, H. Nguyen, M.E. Weksler, Treatment of Old Mice with IL-2 Corrects Dysregulated IL-2 and IL-4 Production, *Int Immunol* (1996) **8** 1009-1015.

[99] D. Frasca, S. Pucci, C. Goso, P. Barattini, S. Barile, C. Pioli, G. Doria, Regulation of Cytokine Production in Aging: Use of Recombinant Cytokines to Upregulate Mitogen-Stimulated Spleen Cells, *Mech Ageing Dev* **93** (1997) 157-169.

[100] G. Candore, G. Di Lorenzo, M. Melluso, γ-Interferon, Interleukin-4 and Interleukin-6 in Vitro Production in Old Subjects, *Autoimmunity* **16** (1993) 275-280.

[101] D. Frasca, L. Adorini, C. Mancini, G. Doria, Reconstitution of T Cell Functions in Aging Mice by Thymosin α1, *Immunopharmacology* **11** (1986) 155-163.

[102] R. Schwab, L.M. Pfeffer, P. Szabo, D. Gamble, C.M. Schnurr, M.E. Weksler, Defective Expression of High Affinity IL-2 Receptors on Activated T Cells from Aged Humans, *Int Immunol* **2** (1990) 239-246.

[103] D. Frasca, L. Guidi, C. Bartoloni, A. Tricerri, M. Vangeli, L. Antico, P.U. Carbonin, A. Errani, G. Doria, Age-Related Modulation of Cytokine Production, IL-2R Expression and Function in a Population of Healthy Subjects (22 to 97 Years), *Mech Ageing Dev* **5** (1994) 3-12.

[104] F.M. Orson, C.K. Saadeh, D.E. Lewis, D.L. Nelson, IL-2 Receptor Expression by T Cells in Aging Humans, *Cell Immunol*, **124** (1989) 278-291.

[105] S.M. Papciack, G.D. Collins, W.H. Adler, Increased Expression of the IFN-γ Gene in Activated T Cells from Old Mice Is Not Due to Age-Related Differences in m-Rna Regulation, Aging, *Immunol Infect Dis* **6** (1995) 107-123.

[106] J. Born, D. Uthgenannt, C. Dodt, D. Nunninghoff, E. Ringvolt, T. Wagner, H.L. Fehm, Cytokine Production and Lymphocyte Subpopulations in Aged Humans. An Assessment during Nocturnal Sleep, *Mech Ageing Dev* **84** (1995) 113-126.

[107] J. Sindermann, A. Kruse, H.J. Frercks, R.M. Schutz, H. Kirchner, Investigations of the Lymphokine System in Elderly Individuals, *Mech Ageing Dev* **70** (1993) 149-159.

[108] C. Franceschi, D. Monti, P. Sansoni, A. Cossarizza, The Immunology of Exceptional Individuals. the Lesson of Centenarians, *Immunol Today* **16** (1995) 12-16.

EUCAMBIS: Immunology and Ageing in Europe
G. Pawelec (Ed.)
IOS Press, 2000

Age-related increases in DNA damage and mutations in T cells in vivo and in vitro: contributors to alterations in T cell-mediated immune responses ?

Yvonne BARNETT[1], Caitriona KING[2], Heather BRISTOW-CRAIG[1], Caroline WARNOCK[1], Paul HYLAND[1], Eddie GILLESPIE[3], Maeve REA[4], Derek MIDDLETON[5], Martin CURRAN[5], Graham PAWELEC[6] and Christopher BARNETT[1].

[1]*Cancer and Ageing Research Group, University of Ulster, Coleraine, County Londonderry, Northern Ireland.* [2] *Department of Medicine and Therapeutics, University College Dublin, Mater Misericordiae Hospital, Dublin 7, Republic of Ireland* [3]*School of Mathematics and Computing, University of Ulster, Newtownabbey, County Antrim, Northern Ireland.* [4] *Belfast City Hospital, Belfast, Northern Ireland and* [5]*Northern Ireland Tissue Typing Laboratory, Belfast City Hospital, Belfast, Northern Ireland.* [6]*Tübingen Ageing and Tumour Immunology Group, University of Tübingen Medical School, Germany.*

Abstract

In this article we summarise our research findings on 'age-related' alterations to levels of genetic damage in T cells in vivo and in vitro. Results of a longitudinal study on healthy human subjects of different age groups (35-39, 50-54, 65-69, 75-80 and 90-100 years) has revealed age-related increases in the mean level of genetic damage in T lymphocytes from these groups. We also found considerable inter-individual differences in levels of genetic damage within the various age groups. Several of the 75-80 and 90-100 year old subjects had levels of genetic damage similar to those found in subjects in the 35-39 years age group. Where an age-related increase in levels of genetic damage was observed this was accompanied by an age-related decline in DNA repair capacity in T lymphocytes. We found similar levels of DNA repair and alterations in levels of certain antioxidants in vivo in those study subjects aged 75-80 years with levels of genetic damage similar to those aged 35-39 years. When we compared in vivo mutant frequencies at the hprt gene locus within T lymphocytes taken from the same subjects in 1992 and 1997 we saw considerable variation at the individual subject level in changes to mutant frequency occurring over this 5 year timespan. To begin to examine the causes and effects of age-related increases in genetic damage in T lymphocytes we have determined levels of DNA damage in 3 T cell clones, as a function of their proliferative lifespan in vitro. We have observed increases in levels of DNA damage, including reactive oxygen species (ROS) induced DNA damage, with increase in population doubling number. In addition, approximately 7 days after the T cell clones had ceased increasing in number (replicative senescence) a rapid increase in the number of cells (> 85%) containing > 80% DNA damage in the comet tail, a hallmark of apoptotic cells, was observed. We suggest that an accumulation of genetic damage in T cells in vivo may result in a decline in T cell-mediated immune responses by affecting the ability of T cells to undergo clonal expansion upon antigenic stimulation.

1. Introduction

At the outset of the research investigations described in this paper we were interested to investigate the relationships between the efficacy of defence systems against biomolecule damage in vivo, levels of genetic damage, health status and longevity in humans.

The hypothesis that the basic mechanisms of ageing must be sought in instabilities in the organisation and expression of the genetic material was proposed decades ago [reviewed in 1]. We are constantly exposed to a variety of exogenous and endogenously-derived entities and processes which may alter the structure and function of a wide range of biomolecules, including DNA [2-4]. To counteract potential biomolecule damage, cellular defence mechanisms have evolved and include antioxidant enzymes such as superoxide dismutase, glutathione peroxidase, catalase and caeruloplasmin, together with molecules like uric acid, bilirubin, alpha-tocopherol and ascorbic acid. Despite these defences, biomolecule damage can still occur and repair or removal enzymes (e.g. DNA repair enzymes, proteosome and phospholipase-A2) are required to minimise the extent of biomolecule damage. Increases in levels of DNA damage and mutation in various cells and tissues have been reported to occur with increasing age in humans [recently reviewed in a special issue of Mutation Research DNAging, Ref. 5]. It has been proposed that mutations in essential genes, in association with age-related alterations in proteins, lipids and carbohydrates, can result in the degradation of structural elements within the cells, tissues and organs of the body leading to alterations in physiological function and eventually to the development of disease and death [6-8; Figure 1]. From this it can be suggested that efficient defence systems against biomolecule damage are likely to be an important contributor towards successful ageing. In this paper we will describe the results obtained to date from a longitudinal study of in vivo antioxidant defence systems, DNA damage mutation and DNA repair capacity in lymphocytes taken from healthy humans of different ages (35 - 100 years).

When we found an age-related accumulation of genetic damage in T lymphocytes in apparently healthy humans, we became interested in examining whether such damage could contribute to age-related alterations in T cell-mediated immune responses. T lymphocytes play a major role in the immune response and they have been found to be susceptible to dysregulated function in association with ageing [reviewed in: 9]. Successful immune responses depend upon waves of rapid and extensive clonal expansion to combat primary infection, followed by death of most T cells, survival of memory cells and their later reactivation and further clonal expansion. If T cells from elderly donors function suboptimally at any stage in this process, the overall effectiveness and duration of the immune response would be greatly compromised, as is often the case. We have embarked upon an analysis of the causes and effects of genetic damage on T cell proliferative capacity. To facilitate these investigations we are utilising an established in vitro T cell model [10]. T cell clone cultures manifest finite in vitro lifespans, together with altered immune function during 'ageing' [11, 12]. In this paper we will describe preliminary results of DNA damage levels within T cells as a function of proliferative lifespan in vitro.

2. Materials and Methods

2.1 In vivo antioxidant status, DNA damage, mutation and DNA repair capacity in human lymphocytes as a function of age - Y. Barnett, King, Bristow-Craig, Warnock, Gillespie, Rea, Middleton, Curran, C. Barnett.

To date we have recruited 71 healthy human subjects aged 35-80 years, non-smokers and not on any prescribed medication, and very recently in association with Rea, Curran and Middleton, 25 free-living subjects aged >85 years, some of whom were taking medication. A 50 ml peripheral blood sample was collected by venipuncture into lithium heparin-coated vacutainers^{R} (Becton Dickinson) from each of the study subjects. Mononuclear cells (MNCs) were isolated from whole blood by density gradient centrifugation using Lymphocyte Separation Medium (Flow Laboratories), washed once in

RPMI 1640 (Dutch Modification, Imperial), once in RPMI 1640 and 10% foetal calf serum (FCS; Gibco), then resuspended at 1 x 10^6 cells/ml in RPMI 1640 containing 10% FCS, 4% sodium pyruvate (200µg/ml), 100 U/ml penicillin and 100µg/ml streptomycin (RPMI growth medium). Cultures were then incubated overnight at 37°C in a 5% CO_2; air, humidified atmosphere. Following incubation, non-adhering cells (lymphocytes) were removed, the number of viable lymphocytes counted using a hemocytometer and resuspended at a concentration of 1 x 10^6 cells/ml in RPMI growth medium. The erythrocyte concentrate and plasma fractions were also collected and stored separately at -70°C prior to the determination of in vivo antioxidant levels.

Erythrocyte superoxide dismutase (SOD; EC 1.15.1.1) activity was determined using an automated (Cobas Fara autoanalyser, Roche) technique and a commercially available kit (Ransod, Randox Laboratories) based on the method described by Jones and Suttle [13]. Erythrocyte glutathione peroxidase (GPx; EC 1.11.1.9) activity was measured on the Cobas Fara autoanalyser using a commercial kit (Ransel, Randox Laboratories) based on the method of Paglia and Valentine [14]. Erythrocyte catalase (CAT; EC 1.11.1.6) activity was measured manually using the method of Aebi [15]. Since SOD, GPx and CAT activities are expressed according to the corresponding sample erythrocyte haemoglobin (Hb) concentration, Hb was measured according to the method of Dacie and Lewis [16]. Plasma caeruloplasmin (CPL) was manually measured using the method of Schosinsky et al. [17]. Plasma uric acid was measured using the Cobas Fara autoanalyser and a commercial kit (Roche Diagnostics) based on the method of Barham and Trinder [18]. Plasma bilirubin was measured on the Cobas Fara autoanalyser using a kit obtained from Roche Diagnostics and based on the method of Malloy and Evelyn [19].

Basal levels of DNA damage within lymphocyte samples from subjects aged 35-80 years of age were quantitated using a sandwich ELISA. The ELISA is based on the action of the monoclonal antibody D1B, directed against single-stranded DNA (SS-DNA). Lymphocyte samples were subjected to controlled, partial alkaline unwinding to convert single-strand breaks, double strand breaks and alkali-labile sites into stretches of SS-DNA to which the antibody molecules could subsequently bind. The extent of binding was then assayed by the addition of an alkaline phosphatase-labelled DIB in a sandwich ELISA. The chromogenic substrate, para-nitrophenyl phosphate, was then added and the optical density, proportional to the degree of SS-DNA, was determined using a microtitre plate reader. Full details of the ELISA protocol employed have been described elsewhere [20]. The ability of the lymphocytes from the study subjects (aged 35-80 years) to repair hydrogen peroxide-induced DNA damage was assessed using the ELISA according to the method detailed in [20] and in the legend to Table 2.

The mutant frequency at the hypoxanthine phosphoribosyltransferase (hprt) gene locus in samples of cultured lymphocytes was estimated using a cloning assay. Essentially, 96-well microtiter[R] flat-bottomed plates were inoculated with 1 x 10^4 GM1899A feeder cells (which had been X-ray irradiated [40Gy]) per well and either 3 lymphocytes/well (2 plates per sample for estimation of plating efficiency) or 2 x 10^4 lymphocytes/well (5-8 plates per sample for selection of HPRT- mutant cells). Each well also contained 200µl of growth medium (RPMI 1640 with 10% foetal calf serum, 4% sodium pyruvate [200µg/ml], 100 U/ml penicillin and 100µg/ml streptomycin) supplemented with 200 U/ml interleukin-2 (human recombinant from Eurocetus) and 5µg/ml phytohaemagglutinin (HA15, Wellcome Diagnostics). Mutant selection plates also contained 5 x 10^{-6}M 6-thioguanine. Plates were incubated on a sloped shelf, at 37°C in a 5% CO_2:air, humidified atmosphere. Growing cells formed a crescent when the slope was reversed 24h prior to scoring. After ~15 days the plates were scored visually using an inverted phase contrast microscope. Wells containing 50 colonies were scored as positive. Mutant frequencies were calculated using standard formulae [21].

2.2 Basal levels of DNA damage in human T cell clones as a function of proliferative lifespan in vitro - Y. Barnett, Hyland, Pawelec and C. Barnett

Three peripheral blood-derived T cell clones (340-73, 385-2 and 385-2a) from healthy human subjects were used in this investigation. 385-2 and 385-2a represent the same clonal population. However, the clone was divided into two at ~ 26 population

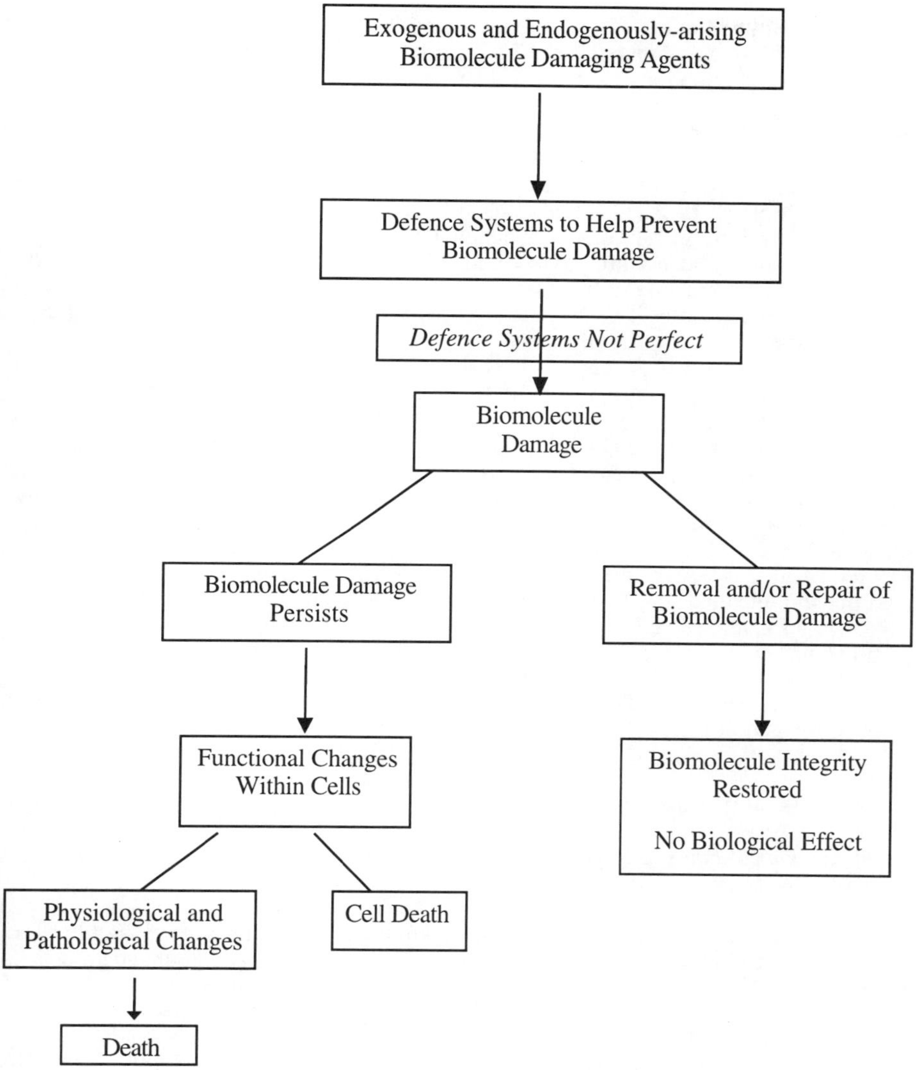

Figure 1: Biomolecule damage, physiological and pathological changes in vivo.
Cellular biomolecules are subject to damage by a wide range of exogenous and endogenously arising entities. Although cellular defence systems exist, which aim to prevent/minimise biomolecule damage, they are not perfect and biomolecule damage still occurs. The accumulation of such biomolecule damage, either alone, or in combination with other age-related changes, can lead to altered physiological function within cells, tissues and organs. Such physiological changes may lead to the onset of pathology and eventually death.

doublings. Both aliquots of the clones were then cultured according to standard procedures, 385-2 was cultured on B-LCL feeder cells, whereas 385-2a was cultured on pooled peripheral blood mononuclear cells up to 35 population doublings. The 3 clones were seeded at a concentration of 2.5×10^5 cells/well in 24-well plates in RPMI 1640 with Glutamax-1 containing 10% FCS, 100 U/ml penicillin, 100μg/ml streptomycin, 40 U/ml recombinant human interleukin-2 (rhIL-2) and 2×10^5 irradiated (80 Gy) RJK feeder cells. The cells were maintained in culture in a seven day cycle. On the fourth day of the cycle fresh IL-2 was added to a final concentration of 40 U/ml and on the seventh day the cells were harvested, viable cells were counted using a hemocytometer and another cycle of culture set up with fresh growth medium and feeder cells. The cell count was used to facilitate the determination of the number of population doublings which the T cells had undergone. The remaining T cells were then cryopreserved prior to determination of levels of DNA damage.

Determination of levels of DNA damage in T cells was performed using the alkaline comet assay according to the method of Singh et al. [22], and with minor modification. Essentially, an aliquot of T cells were embedded in agarose gel on a total of 6 microscope slides and lysed under alkaline conditions. Three of the microscope slides were then treated with endonuclease III (which has both an apurinic/apyrimidinic endonuclease activity and a DNA glycosylase activity which releases pyrimidine residues damaged by ring saturation, fragmentation or ring contraction [23]) in reaction buffer (0.1M KCl, 0.5 mM EDTA, 40 mM HEPES-KOH, 0.2 mg/ml bovine serum albumin, pH 8.0) for 1 h at 37^{0}C. All of the microscope slides were then subjected to electrophoresis at high pH and uncoiled SS-DNA migrated towards the anode faster than double-stranded DNA. Each damaged cell had the appearance of a comet when stained with ethidium bromide and viewed under UV light, with a brightly fluorescent head and a tail whose intensity was related to the number of strand breaks (reported as % DNA in comet tail). Stained slides were analysed using a UV microscope and the Comet 3.0 analysis program (Kinetic Imaging, Liverpool).

3. Results and Discussion

3.1 In vivo antioxidant status, DNA damage, mutation and DNA repair capacity in human lymphocytes as a function of age

Figure 2 summarises the results obtained following determination of basal levels of DNA damage within lymphocytes from healthy human subjects in the four age groups 35-39, 50-54, 65-69 and 75-80 years. We found an age-related increase in basal levels of DNA damage from 35-69 years. These data are in agreement with Hartwig and Korner [24] and Turner et al. [25] also showed an age-related increase in DNA single strand breaks within human lymphocytes. At the group level, there was significantly more DNA damage in the lymphocytes of subjects in the 65-69 years age group, compared to the 35-39 years age group (Student's t-test; $p = 0.0013$, at 5% level of significance). However, the mean basal level of DNA damage for the 75-80 years age group was not significantly different from that of the 35-39 years age group ($p = 0.65$), and was significantly lower than that observed for the 65-69 years age group ($p = 0.004$). There was considerable inter-individual variation in basal levels of DNA damage within the different age groups (levels of DNA damage within lymphocytes from individual subjects have been documented elsewhere [20, 26]). Such variation is not surprising since a variety of dietary, lifestyle and genetic factors (including in vivo antioxidant status) can affect DNA damage levels in vivo.

Other groups have reported an apparent age-related increase in mutant frequency at the hprt locus [reviewed in 27]. The mean values obtained for in vivo mutant frequency at the hprt locus for the different age groups are illustrated in Figure 3. We observed an age-related increase in mean age group mutant frequency values, with the mean values for the 65-69 and 90-100 years age group being significantly greater than that for the 35-39 years age group ($p < 0.05$). The mean 75-80 years age group mutant frequency was not significantly different from that of the 35-39 years age group ($t = 1.25$, $p = 0.11$). The reason for the low mean group mutant frequency within the 75-80 years age group remains

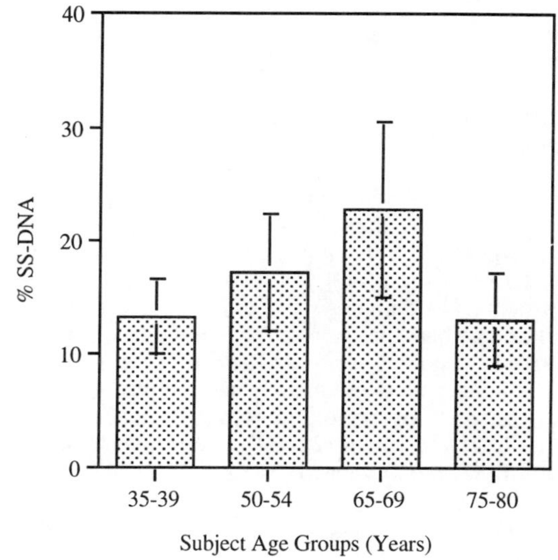

Figure 2: Mean Age Group Basal Levels of DNA Damage in Lymphocytes.
Basal levels of DNA damage in lymphocytes taken from healthy humans of different ages were determined using an ELISA (see Materials and Methods). The mean basal levels of DNA damage for the age groups were: 35-39 years, 13.3±3.3, n = 15; 50-54 years, 17.2±5.2, n = 5; 65-69 years, 22.8±7.8, n = 11; 75-80 years, 13.1±4.1, n = 18.

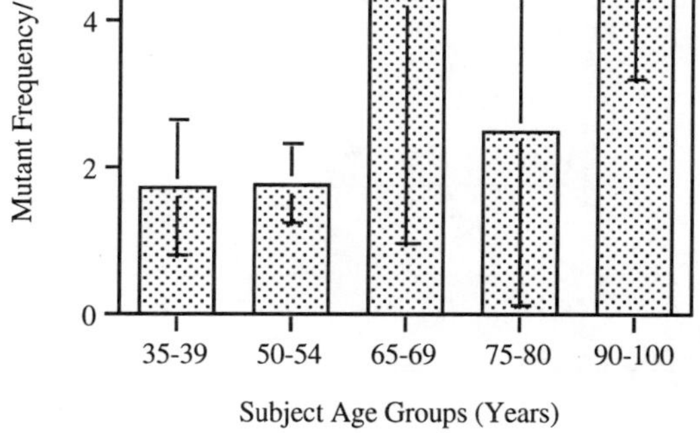

Figure 3: Mean Age Group Mutant Frequencies.
Mutant frequencies at the hprt gene locus in lymphocytes from healthy humans within different age groups were determined using a clonal assay (see Materials and Methods). Mean age group mutant frequencies were: 35-39 years, 1.73±0.92, n = 20; 50-54 years, 1.79±0.55, n = 18; 65-69 years, 4.33±3.35, n = 17; 75-80 years, 2.48±2.36, n = 16; >85 years, 5.51±2.31, n = 25.

to be elucidated. This group may represent a subpopulation of individuals who have 'aged successfully', having reached the average life expectancy, they were all still healthy and not on prescribed medication. A number of the subjects > 90 years of age were on some form of prescribed medication at the time of sampling. None of the medication has been reported to have any genotoxic effects in vivo, and so did not contribute to the levels of genetic damage measured. We observed considerable inter-individual differences in mutant frequency, from 65 years onwards. Within each of the three older age groups there were individuals with very low mutant frequency values, comparable to those obtained for subjects aged < 39 years, whereas the in vivo mutant frequency values of others were significantly higher than those of the 35-39 year olds. In vivo levels of mutation will depend upon the way in which DNA damage is processed. DNA damage may be repaired, tolerated, cause cell death or may become fixed to form mutations. It is likely that efficient processing of DNA damage to restore its original structure will result in a slower rate of accumulation of mutation in vivo, with consequent beneficial physiological outcome.

Protection of biomolecules by antioxidants has been described as a longevity determinant process, so too has DNA repair [28, 29]. In our investigations we assessed in vivo antioxidant status and DNA repair capacity within the subjects aged 35-80 years to see how these defence endpoints compared with the in vivo levels of genetic damage. Table 1 shows that there were significant increases in levels of CAT, CPL and GPx within the 75-80 year old age group, compared to the other age groups. Increased in vivo levels of reactive oxygen species (ROS) have been reported for some [30, 31] studies. We suggest that the increased levels of CAT, CPL and GPx within the 75-80 year old age group may be a protective response to increased levels of ROS in vivo in this age group, compared to the other age groups examined within our study. The ability to mount and maintain such a protective response is likely to be an important contributor to maintaining biomolecule structure and function in vivo. Conflicting data on age-related changes to DNA repair capacity have been reported, and are likely to be due to the cell and tissue type under analysis, as well as the methods used to estimate DNA repair capacity [reviewed in 20].

Table 1: Significant alterations in levels of caeruloplasmin, catalase and glutathione peroxidase within subjects aged 75-80 years

Antioxidant / Age Group (years)	Caeruloplasmin (U/l)	Catalase (k/gHb)	Glutathione peroxidase (U/gHb)
35-39 n = 20	147±45	67±24	37±10
50-54 n = 18	103±49	49±20	43±10
65-69 n = 17	122±63	58±49	40±10
75-80 n = 16	199±46	262±73	92±15

The results of our investigations to determine in vivo levels of the antioxidants, bilirubin, superoxide dismutatse and uric acid, did not reveal any age-related changes in levels (results are detailed elsewhere [26]). However, as the results in the table above show there were significant increases (ANOVA) in the levels of caeruloplasmin ($F = 16.13$; $p = 0.00$), catalase ($F = 84.11$; $p = 0.00$) and glutathione peroxidase ($F = 120.95$; $p = 0.00$) within subjects aged 75-80 years, compared with the other age groups. Results represent mean values± SD.

Table 2 shows levels of hydrogen peroxide induced DNA damage remaining 90 minutes after treatment of lymphocytes from subjects aged 35-80 years. Our results show that there was an age-related decline in DNA repair capacity between 35 and 69 years. However, the extent of DNA repair in lymphocytes from the 75-80 year age group was similar to that of the 35-39 year olds. Thus, the DNA repair capacity parallels the in vivo levels of genetic damage within our study subjects. Our results highlight the importance of antioxidant status and DNA repair capacity in the maintenance of genomic stability in vivo. The results of earlier studies on centenarians by Franceschi et al. [32, 33] also led them to tentatively suggest a relationship between increased genomic stability, efficient in vivo defence systems and longevity.

Table 2: Levels of DNA damage remaining 90 minutes following treatment of lymphocytes from subjects in the 35-39, 50-54, 65-69 and 75-80 years age groups with hydrogen peroxide

Age Group (years) /	35-39 n = 15	50-54 n = 5	65-69 n = 11	75-80 n = 18
Levels of DNA damage (%SS-DNA)	5.2±3.9	7.3±2.3	10.9±5.6	4.8±4.4

Lymphocytes were treated on ice (to minimise DNA repair) for 1 hour with 200μM hydrogen peroxide; thereafter they were maintained in culture at 37°C and aliquots of cells were removed over a 480 min time course for determination of levels of DNA damage using an ELISA. The results in this table show an age-related increase (from 35-69 years) in the amount of DNA damage remaining 90 min following treatment. Levels of DNA damage remaining after 90 min in the 75-80 year old lymphocyte samples were not statistically different from levels within lymphocytes from the 35-39 year olds ($p = 0.87$; Student's t-test). The results obtained for levels of DNA damage remaining at the other sampling points showed a similar pattern of change (results not shown). From the data obtained we inferred an age-related decline (35-69 years) in the ability of lymphocytes to repair hydrogen peroxide-induced DNA damage. However, DNA repair capacity in the 75-80 year old subjects was similar to that of the 35-39 year olds, in parallel with similar levels of genetic damage in vivo for the two different age groups.

We have embarked upon a longitudinal study to further investigate the complex inter-relationships between in vivo defence systems, diet and lifestyle factors, levels of genetic damage and health status within our study subjects. When we compared individual subject mutant frequency values from subjects in the 50-54 and 65-69 years age group in 1992 with those obtained for the same subjects following a second blood sampling in 1997 (Figures 4 and 5) we found that the mean group mutant frequency for subjects in the younger of the two age groups had increased significantly from 1.79±0.55/ 10^6 cells in 1992 to 3.77±1.36/ 10^6 cells in 1997 (Student's t-test, $p < 0.001$), whereas the mean group mutant frequency for the older age group (all subjects healthy and not on prescribed medication) did not change over the five year period (4.33±3.35/ 10^6 cells in 1992, 4.56±1.06/ 10^6 cells in 1997). Mutant frequency values increased over the 5 year period within the majority of the younger individuals. There was much more heterogeneity in the relative changes to mutant frequency over the 5 year period within subjects from the older age group. From these results we suggest that if a subject is to remain healthy in later years it becomes increasingly important to ensure that levels of biomolecule damage (exemplified within our study by levels of genetic damage) are kept in check. It will be interesting to follow the various damage and defence endpoints within these study subjects as they age and see how they correlate with health status and longevity. The results of such an investigation may provide us with a set of biomarkers indicative of an individual's capacity to age successfully.

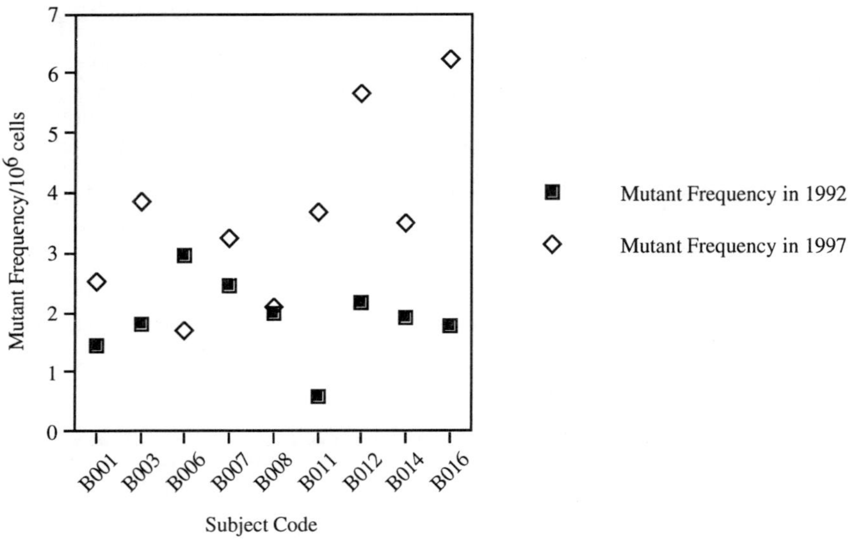

Figure 4: In Vivo Mutant Frequencies in Lymphocytes from Individual Healthy Subjects Sampled in 1992 and 1997.

The mutant frequency at the hprt gene locus in lymphocytes taken from healthy humans in the 50-54 years age group was determined in 1992. To enable investigation of age-related changes to in vivo mutant load, blood samples were collected from these same individuals in 1997 and the mutant frequency at the hprt gene locus determined.

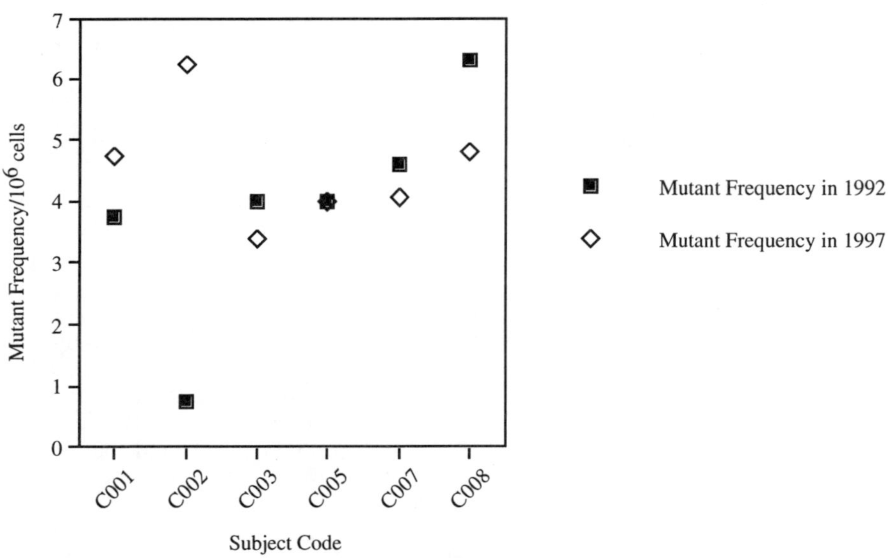

Figure 5: In Vivo Mutant Frequencies in Lymphocytes from Healthy Subjects Sampled in 1992 and 1997.

The mutant frequency at the hprt gene locus in lymphocytes taken from healthy humans in the 65-69 years age group was determined in 1992. To enable investigation of age-related changes to in vivo mutant load, blood samples were collected from these same individuals in 1997 and the mutant frequency at the hprt gene locus determined.

3.2 Basal levels of DNA damage in human T cell clones as a function of proliferative lifespan in vitro

Could DNA damage and mutation lead to alterations in T cell proliferative capacity and thus to altered T cell-mediated immune responses in vivo ? The studies of Franceschi et al. [32, 33] showed not only a tendency for increased genomic stability in the T cells of centenarians, but they also established that centenarians have relatively efficient immune responses [reviewed in 34]. This implies a relationship between the efficiency of the T cell-mediated immune response and genomic stability. To facilitate further investigation of the causes and effects of genetic damage accumulation within T cells we have embarked upon an examination of levels of genetic damage and proliferative status of T cell clones in vitro. Proliferative lifespans and replicative senescence have been extensively studied in other tissues, especially fibroblasts. The term replicative senescence describes the characteristic of all normal somatic cells to undergo a finite and predictable number of cell divisions in vitro before reaching an irreversible state of growth arrest (so-called 'Hayflick limit', [35]). Recent studies have demonstrated that in Down's syndrome (a condition of accelerated ageing) and in centenarians, T cells with characteristics of senescent cultured cells exist in vivo [reviewed in 36]. Figure 6 illustrates the first results obtained on the analysis of levels of DNA damage as a function of proliferative lifespan for the 3 T cell clones. The results obtained for 385-2 and 385-2a were virtually identical. This confirms that the use of the different feeder cells for 9 population doublings did not affect the genetic damage load or ability to respond to genetic damage within these clones. The levels of DNA damage obtained using the basic comet assay did not show any significant alterations with increase in population doubling number for any of the clones. However, we found that, on average, 7 days after the T cell clones had ceased increasing in number (had reached apparent replicative senescence) the majority of T cells had levels of DNA damage consistent with those of apoptotic cells (> 80% DNA in comet tail [37]; data not shown). We are now interested to establish the role of accumulated DNA damage in the

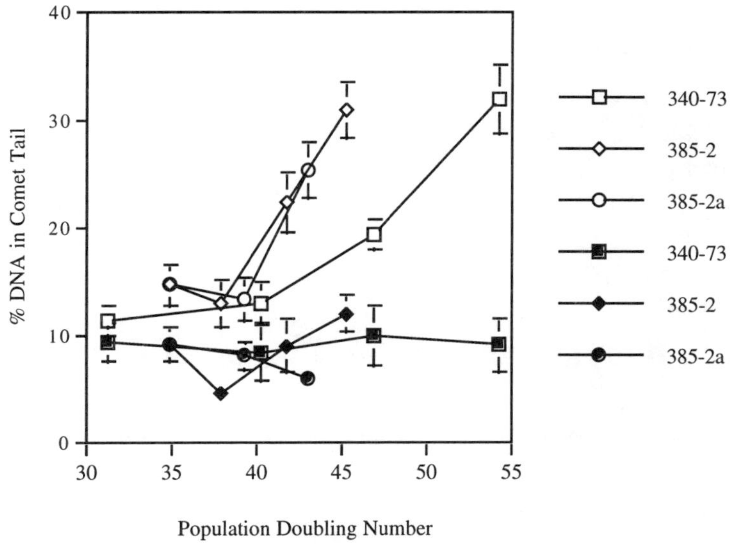

Figure 6: Levels of DNA Damage in T Cell Clones as a Function of Their Lifespan In Vitro. Levels of DNA damage in 3 T cell clones were determined using the basic comet assay (results illustrated with filled symbols) and a modified comet assay (results illustrated with open symbols) at various timepoints during their lifespan in vitro.

initiation of replicative senescence within the T cells in vitro. The 3 T cell clones were cultured in an atmosphere containing 20% oxygen. Under such conditions, ROS are likely to be a major contributor to DNA damage. Indeed, at sites of inflammatory foci and as a consequence of normal physiological processes in vivo, ROS and reactive nitrogen species are likely to represent a major source of damaging entities for T cells [4, 38, 39]. When we compared the level of DNA damage within a sample of a T cell clone at a defined population doubling using the basic alkaline comet assay and compared this with the level of DNA damage within the same sample, the DNA of which had been subjected to treatment with endonuclease III (cleaves at many of the types of lesions produced by ROS [23, 40-43] prior to the comet assay, we found a substantial increase in levels of DNA damage after endonuclease III treatment.

How then might genetic damage affect T cell-mediated immune responses ? That effective T cell-mediated immunity is dependent upon the amplification of the response by clonal expansion requires T cells to be efficiently stimulated by the relevant antigens and then to undergo numerous rounds of cell division in order to generate appropriate responses. A normal cell can respond in a number of ways to DNA damage: cell cycle arrest and/or repair of the DNA damage [44], tolerate the DNA damage and continue to replicate, or undergo apoptosis in response to critical levels of DNA damage [45]. In addition, cells containing mutations in any number of genes for normal cellular metabolism may be selected against in vivo. T cells containing such mutations would perhaps have a reduced capacity for proliferation, be unable to proliferate given the appropriate stimuli, or may not be viable. For example, human T lymphocytes which contain a mutation in the *hprt* gene have reduced proliferation rates in vitro [46] and appear to be selected against in vivo [47]. Thus, genetic damage has the potential to prevent or reduce the proliferation of T cells following antigenic stimulation. Further understanding of the causes of genetic damage, and the mechanisms through which it exerts its effects on T cell proliferation may enable a contribution to interventive strategies aimed at maintaining the efficacy of the immune response as we age.

4. Acknowledgements

The authors wish to express sincere thanks to: the study subjects who participated in the investigations described above; Dr Andrew Collins, The Rowett Research Institute, Aberdeen, Scotland for the kind gift of Endonuclease III; The EU (under the auspices of EUCAMBIS), DevR Funding and the Department of Health and Social Services, Northern Ireland and the VERUM Foundation for providing financial support for these investigations.

5. References

[1] P.E. Slagboom and J. Vijg, Genetic instability and aging: theories, facts and future perspectives, *Genome* **31** (1989) 373-385.

[2] T. Sugimura, Successful use of short-term tests for academic purposes: Their use in identification of new environmental carcinogens with posible risk for humans. *Mutation Research* **205** (1988) 33-39.

[3] B.A. Freeman and J.D. Crapo, Biology of disease, free radicals and tissue injury, *Laboratory Investigation*, **47** (1982) 412-426.

[4] T. Lindahl, Instability and decay of the primary structure of DNA, *Nature* **362** (1993) 709-715.

[5] Somatic mutations and aging: cause or effect ?, *Mutation Research* - DNAging section, special issue **338** (1995) 1-234.

[6] R.E. Pacifici and K.J.A. Davies, Protein, lipid and DNA repair systems in oxidative stress; the free radical theory revisited, *Gerontology* **37** (1991) 166-180.

[7] S.L. Mera, Senescence and pathology in ageing, *Medical Laboratory Science* **49** (1992) 271-282.

[8] Y.A. Barnett, How and why we age ?. In: J.M. Allen, Y.A. Barnett, F. Gibson, F. and P.G. McKenna (eds.), Celebrating Age. ISBN 1 85628 589 8 Avebury Press, Aldershot, 1995 pp. 78-92.

[9] G. Pawelec, E. Remarque, Y. Barnett and R. Solana, T cells and ageing, *Frontiers in Bioscience* **3** (1998) 59-99. (www.bioscience.org)

[10] G. Pawelec, Cloning and propagation of human T lymphocytes. In: G. Gallagher, R.C. Rees and C.W. Reynolds (eds.),Tumour Immunobiology: A Practical Approach. Oxford University Press, 1992, pp. 131-141.

[11] G. Pawelec, Molecular and cell biological studies of ageing and their application to considerations of T lymphocyte immunosenescence, *Mechanisms of Ageing and Development* **79** (1995) 1-32.

[12] M. Adibzadeh, H. Pohla, A. Rehbein and G. Pawelec, Long-term culture of monoclonal human T-lymphocytes: models for immunosenescence. *Mechanisms of Ageing and Development* **8 3** (1995) 171-183.

[13] D.G. Jones and N.F. Suttle, Some effects of copper deficiency on leucocyte function in sheep and cattle, *Research in Veterinary Science* **31** (1981) 151-156.

[14] D.E. Paglia and W.N. Valentine, Characteristics of erythrocyte glutathione peroxidase, *Journal of Laboratory and Clinical Medicine* **70** (1967) 158.

[15] A.B.H. Aebi, Catalase. In: R. Bergmeyer (ed.), Methods of Enzymatic Analysis, Vol. 2, Academic Press, New York, 1974, pp. 643-684.

[16] J.V. Dacie, J.V. and S.M Lewis. In: Practical Haematology, 5th ed., Churchill and Livingstone, 1975, pp. 30-37.

[17] K.H. Schosinsky, H.P. Lehmann and M.F. Beller, Measurement of caeruloplasmin activity in serum by use of O-dianesidinedihydrochloride, *Clinical Chemistry* **20** (1974)1556-1563.

[18] D. Barham and P. Trinder, Improved colour reagent for determination of blood glucose by oxidase system, *Analyst* **97** (1972) 142-145.

[19] H.T. Malloy and K.A. Evelyn, Determination of bilirubin with photoelectric calorimetry, *Journal of Biological Chemistry* **119** (1937) 481-490.

[20] Y.A. Barnett and C.M. King, An investigation of in vivo antioxidant status, mutation and DNA repair capacity in human lymphocytes as a function of age, *Mutation Research* **338** (1995) 115-128.

[21] C.M. King, E.S. Gillespie, P.G. McKenna and Y.A. Barnett, An investigation of mutation as a function of age in humans, *Mutation Research* **316** (1994) 79-90.

[22] N.P. Singh, M.T. McCoy, R.R. Tice and E.L. Schneider, A simple technique for quantitation of low levels of DNA damage in individual cells, *Experimental Cell Research* **175** (1988) 184-191.

[23] H. Asahara, P.M. Wistort, J.F. Bank, R.H. Bakerian and R.P. Cunningham, Purification and characterisation of E. coli Endonuclease III from the cloned nth gene. *Biochemistry* **28** (1989) 4444-4449.

[24] M. Hartwig and I.J. Korner, Age-related changes in DNA unwinding and repair in human peripheral lymphocytes, *Mechanisms of Ageing and Development* **39** (1987) 73-78.

[25] D.R. Turner, A.A. Morley, R.S. Seshadri and J.R. Sorrell, Age related variations in human lymphocytes DNA, *Mechanisms of Ageing and Development* **17** (1981) 305-309.

[26] C.M. King, H.E. Bristow-Craig, E.S. Gillespie and Y.A. Barnett, In vivo antioxidant status, DNA damage, mutation and DNA repair capacity in cultured lymphocytes from healthy 75-80 year old humans, *Mutation Research* **377** (1997) 137-147.

[27] J. Cole and T.R. Skopek, Somatic mutant frequency, mutation rates and mutational spectra in the human population in vivo, *Mutation Research* **304** (1994) 33-105.

[28] R.G. Cutler, Antioxidants, aging and longevity. In: W.A. Pryor, (Ed.) Free Radicals in Biology Volume VI. Academic Press, New York. 1984, pp. 371-428.

[29] R.W. Hart and R.B. Setlow, Correlation between deoxyribonucleic acid excision repair and lifespan in a number of mammalian species, *Proceedings of the National Academy of Sciences (USA)*, **71** (1974) 2169-2173.

[30] M. Sagai and T. Ichinose, Age-related changes in lipid peroxidation as measured by ethane, ethylene, butane and pentane in respired gases by rats, *Life Sciences* **27** (1980) 731-738.

[31] E.R. Stadtman, Protein oxidation and aging, *Science* **257** (1992) 1220-1224.

[32] C. Franceschi, D. Monti, A. Cossarizza, F. Fagnoni, G. Passeri and P. Sansoni, Aging, longevity, and cancer: Studies in Down's syndrome and centenarians, *Annals of the New York Academy of Sciences* **621** (1991) 428-440.

[33] C. Franceschi, D. Monti, M.R. Scarfi, O. Zeni, P. Temperani, G. Emilia, P. Sansoni, M.B. Lioi, C.A. Troiano, S. Salvioli and A. Cossarizza, Genomic stability and aging: Studies in centenarians and in patients with Down's syndrome. *Annals of the New York Academy of Sciences* **663** (1992) 4-16.

[34] C. Franceschi, D. Monti, P. Sansoni and A. Cossarizza, The immunology of exceptional individuals: the lesson of centenarians, *Immunology Today* **12** (1995)12-16.

[35] L. Hayflick and P.S. Moorehead, The serial cultivation of human diploid cell strains, *Experimental Cell Research* **25** (1961) 585-621.

[36] R.B. Effros and G. Pawelec, Replicative senescence of T cells: does the Hayflick Limit lead to immune exhaustion? *Immunology Today* **18** (1997) 450-454.

[37] B.E. Nelms, R. Moravec and T. Riss, Measuring apoptosis in individual cells with the comet assay, *Promega Notes Magazine* **64** (1998) 13-16.

[38] Z. Metzger, J.T. Hoffeld and J.J. Oppenheim, Macrophage-mediated suppression: I Evidence for participation of both hydrogen peroxide and prostaglandins in suppression of murine lymphocyte proliferation, *Journal of Immunology* **124** (1980) 983-988.

[39] S.H. Gregory, E.J. Wing, R.A. Hoffman and R.L. Simmons, Reactive nitrogen intermediates suppress the primary immunologic response to *Listeria*, *Journal of Immunology* **150** (1993) 2901-2909.

[40] Y.W.Kow and S.S. Wallace, Exonuclease III recognises urea residues in oxidised DNA, *Proceedings of the National Academy of Sciences (USA)* **82** (1985) 8354-8358.

[41] S.B. Farr, R. D'Ari and D. Touati, Oxygen-dependent mutagenesis in *Escherichia coli* lacking superoxide dismutase, *Proceedings of the National Academy of Sciences (USA)* **83** (1986) 8268-8272.

[42] O.I. Arouma, B. Halliwell, E. Gajewski and M. Dizdaroglu, Damage to the bases in DNA induced by hydrogen peroxide and ferric ion chelates, *Journal of Biological Chemistry* **264** (1989) 20509-20512.

[43] S. Shibutani, M. Takeshita and A.P. Grollman, Insertion of specific bases during DNA synthesis past the oxidation damaged base 8-oxodG, *Nature (London)* **349** (1991) 431-434.

[44] L.H. Hartwell and M.B. Kastan, Cell cycle control and cancer, *Science* (1994) 1821-1828.

[45] M.L. Smith and A.J. Fornace, Mammalian DNA damage-inducible genes associated with growth arrest and apoptosis, *Mutation Research* **340** (1996) 109-124.

[46] A. Podlutsky, T. Bastlova and B. Lambert, Reduced proliferation rate of hypoxanthine-phosphoribosyl transferase mutant human T-lymphocytes in vitro. *Environmental and Molecular Mutagenesis* **28** (1996) 13-18.

[47] J.L. Dempsey, A.A. Morley, R.S. Seshadri, Detection of the carrier state for an X-linked disorder, the Lesch-Nyhan syndrome, by the use of lymphocyte cloning. Hum. Genet., 64 (1983) 288-290.

Influenza vaccination in elderly people

E.J. Remarque and I.A. de Bruijn
Section of Gerontology and Geriatrics, Leiden University Medical Centre, building 1 P-3 Q, PO box 9600, 2300 RC Leiden, The Netherlands

Abstract. Influenza is an important cause of morbidity and mortality in the elderly. Influenza vaccine has been shown to successfully reduce influenza- and pneumonia-associated hospitalizations and deaths, but the antibody induction by influenza vaccines is not always optimal in the elderly. The lower serological efficacy of influenza vaccines that is often observed in the elderly may be due to a multitude of factors. In this review we will discuss some of these factors. These include health status and previous exposures to influenza viruses. In addition, we will discuss possibilities to improve antibody responses and the effects of annually repeated vaccinations.

1. Introduction

Influenza is an infectious disease in mammals and birds caused by influenza viruses. In man, the impact of influenza can be devastating: in 1918 - 1919 the world was struck by a pandemic of influenza, causing more than 20 million deaths world-wide. This "Spanish flu" at the end of the First World War caused more deaths than four years of war (1). Although not as devastating as in 1918 - 1919, influenza remains an important cause of morbidity and mortality (2-5).

Most of the serious morbidity and mortality caused by influenza occurs in the elderly (3,6,7). In the Netherlands with a population of 15 million people, 1,000 to 4,000 deaths each year are attributed to influenza and influenza-related complications. Of these influenza-related deaths, 95% occur amongst those older than 60 years of age (3,4). The risk for influenza-related mortality increases with advancing age, with approximately 50% of all influenza-related deaths occurring amongst people older than 80 years of age (3,4). The incidence of pneumonia associated with influenza also increases sharply with advancing age (8-10). Hospitalisation and the occurrence of influenza-related complications, like pneumonia, can cause loss of independence for previously healthy elderly, resulting in dependency on health care and social care (11).

Pneumonia is often regarded as "the old man's best friend", suggesting that only frail elderly die from complications associated with an influenza infection. This assumption, however, is probably not true because a period of high influenza morbidity is not followed by a dip in mortality rates (12). In addition, Glezen *et al.* demonstrated that 40% of influenza-related hospital admissions were not of patients belonging to risk groups (13). A similar observation was made by Barker and Mullooly, who reported that 50% of pneumonia and influenza-related deaths occurred in persons previously in good health or in chronically ill, but stable patients (10).

The greying of the population is the most characteristic demographic change of the 20th century. Lower birth rates and an increased life expectancy have resulted in a decreased population growth and greying of the population. As a consequence, the proportion of the Dutch population aged 65 and over can be expected to increase from 13% in 1990 to 23% in

2050 (14). Moreover the proportion of the population aged 85 and over is expected to increase from 1.2% in 1990 to 3.5% in 2050 (14). Due to the increased proportion of elderly in the population, the impact of influenza can be expected to increase in the near future, resulting in an increased medical and economical burden.

A recently experienced natural influenza infection is an effective way to prevent, or reduce, the severity of subsequent infections with drifted influenza viruses (5,15,16). Influenza should however be prevented in the elderly, because it causes severe morbidity and excess mortality in this age group. The protection induced by an influenza infection can be mimicked by influenza vaccination, thus inducing immunity without causing disease. Influenza can also be prevented by medication, but the drugs available, Amantadine and Rimantadine, are only effective against influenza A viruses. In addition, these drugs can cause severe side effects and viral resistance can abolish the effects of medication (17-22). Currently, new drugs are being developed that are effective against type A and B viruses (23). These drugs show promising effects in *in vitro* tests and in animal models, but up to now, vaccination is the only feasible strategy to prevent influenza in the elderly.

The protective efficacy of the vaccine in the elderly depends on the immunogenicity of the vaccine and on sufficient antigenic match between the vaccine and epidemic viruses (24). Thus, the vaccine can be efficacious in preventing influenza-related morbidity and mortality in some cases (8,25-32), whereas in other cases the vaccine may fail to protect (33-39). As the antigenic make up of influenza viruses changes frequently and antibody titres decrease in time, there is a need for annually repeated influenza vaccinations. However, there have been reports indicating that annual revaccination may be less efficacious than single vaccinations (40).

In this chapter we will describe our research on the efficacy of influenza vaccination in elderly people. There are three main issues, viz. The influence of age on the seroresponse and T cell parameters, the influence of health status and finally the influence of annually repeated influenza vaccinations.

2. Age influence on the seroresponse to influenza vaccine

The changes in the immune system during ageing are diverse and may influence the antibody response to influenza vaccine. During ageing, primary T-cell dependent antibody responses decline, whereas secondary antibody responses are relatively conserved. In the case of influenza viruses, some antigenic characteristics change, while others are conserved. Thus the response to influenza virus may be a combination of primary and secondary immune responses.

The influence of age on the antibody response following influenza vaccination was investigated by comparing antibody responses in optimal healthy young (JUNIEURS) with those in optimal healthy elderly (SENIEURS). HI and IgG antibody responses to the influenza A (H1N1) vaccine strains were lower in healthy elderly SENIEURS as compared to healthy young JUNIEURS (41-43). A group of elderly subjects did not produce Hemaggluitination Inhibiting (HI) antibody to the H1N1 vaccine strain, but produced antibody to the closely related A/Singapore/6/86 H1N1 strain, which was not contained in the vaccine (41). In addition, the antibody produced by this group of elderly neutralized A/Taiwan/1/86-induced viral cytotoxicity *in vitro* (41). The observation that HI antibody responses to closely related H1N1 strains differs is in agreement with previous findings by Pyhälä *et al.* and these differences in responsiveness to H1N1 strains may be due to age-related differences in priming (44). This age-related altered antibody response to H1N1 strains may have consequences for the protection induced by the vaccine.

By contrast, antibody responses to the influenza A H3N2 strains were similar for both age groups (41-43). Moreover, IgA responses to the H3N2 vaccine strain were higher in the SENIEURS as compared to the JUNIEURS (41). Thus the age-related declined immune response was influenza strain-related and when present, it was mostly confined to the IgG isotype (41). The HI data are in agreement with previous reports (45,46), where a strain-related declined antibody response was observed in healthy elderly subjects.

One could expect that age-related differences at the helper T cell level may explain age-related differences in the antibody response (47,48). Helper T cells from SENIEURS were functionally competent, since the proliferation and IL 2 production of helper T cells after mitogenic stimulation was comparable for SENIEURS and JUNIEURS. Moreover, IL-4 production was higher in the elderly (48).

The number of helper T cells with naive phenotype was negatively correlated with *in vivo* anti-influenza antibody response in JUNIEURS only, whereas the number of helper T cells with memory phenotype was positively correlated with *in vivo* anti-influenza antibody response in both age groups (47). Age-related differences in the composition of the helper T cell compartment however, did not explain age-related differences in antibody responses (47), suggesting that other (antigen specific) factors may be responsible for the declined antibody response to some influenza strains.

The combination of the declined antibody response to some strains (41) and the functional competence of the T cell compartment in the SENIEURS (47,48) makes it tempting to speculate that the age-related differences in antibody response may be due to differences in previous exposures: the original antigenic sin. Thus, the altered response of the SENIEURS (41) to the A/Taiwan/1/86 (H1N1) strain, could be due to the presence of antibodies directed against previous variants of the H1N1 subtype. These antibodies may have interfered with antibody formation against the vaccine strain. This idea is supported by experimental data by McElhaney *et al.* (45). They found that antibody levels to previous H1N1 strains were higher in the elderly as compared to the young.

Because a whole virus vaccine was used in these studies, helper T cells specific for internal proteins may have provided a substantial part of the required T cell help. Since these helper T cells are cross-reactive within one influenza type, differences at the T cell level are less likely to be an explanation for the strain-related declined antibody response in the elderly, although antigen-specific defects at the T helper cell level can not be completely excluded. Additionally, helper T cells specific for conserved regions of the surface glycoproteins may also have provided T cell help. The observation that age-related differences in the composition of the helper T cell compartment do not provide an explanation for the lower antibody response to influenza vaccine is in agreement with previous findings (45).

3. The influence of health status on the antibody response.

The prevalence of various diseases is increased in the elderly and these diseases may affect the functions of the immune system. Therefore the influence of functional disability, disease and use of medication as measures of health status on the humoral immune response to influenza vaccine was investigated.

Elderly patients with ADL (Activities of Daily Living) disabilities had lower postvaccination titres to all influenza vaccine antigens (49). The results consistently demonstrate a correlation between physical disabilities, as determined by ADL, and the humoral immune response to influenza vaccine. A remarkable observation was that the influence of ADL score on antibody levels was in the same order of magnitude for all strains investigated (49). The observation that health status can influence the immune response to influenza vaccine is in agreement with Gross *et al.*, although they only found a correlation between health status and one vaccine component (50).

Since the antibody response in elderly nursing home patients was negatively influenced by functional disability, vaccination strategies have to be developed to improve vaccine efficacy in these patients. Moreover, the declined immune response that occurs in ADL disabled elderly patients after vaccination may also occur in case of an influenza infection; hence ADL disability should be considered to be a risk factor for influenza and influenza-related complications.

In healthy SENIEUR elderly, strain-specific differences occurred in the HI and IgG antibody response (41). In addition, the proportion of IgA antibody relative to the total amount of antibody was higher for all strains in SENIEURS. By contrast, health status, as determined by ADL, influenced the immune response to all strains investigated. This suggests the presence of at least three factors that may influence the antibody response to influenza vaccine in the elderly. First, differences in priming and previous exposures to influenza viruses, second, immunosenescence and finally, disease influences.

4. Improvement of antibody responses to influenza vaccine in the elderly

The antibody response to influenza vaccine is decreased in elderly nursing home residents (49). Since it was reported that immune responsiveness in non-SENIEURS to primary T cell-dependent antigens can be enhanced by increasing the antigen dose (51), the possible beneficial effects of an increased antigen dose on the antibody response to influenza vaccine were investigated (52,53).

The effects of antigen dose on the immunoglobulin (sub)class distribution to the A/Sichuan/2/87 strain (H3N2) were investigated (52). At a 10 μg dose, IgG, IgG_1 and HI responses were twofold lower in the elderly as compared to the young. A 20 μg dose increased the IgG, IgG_1 and HI levels in the elderly to the levels in the young and the IgA_1 to significantly higher levels than in the young. A 60 μg dose increased antibody levels in the young, but did not further increase the response in the elderly. The subclass distribution of the anti-influenza antibodies as observed in the elderly (52), was recently confirmed by Powers *et al.* (54).

In addition, the effects of age and antigen dose on the immunoglobulin isotype distribution to the A/Taiwan/1/86 (H1N1) strain were investigated (53). At a 10 μg dose, HI and IgG responses were lower in the elderly. IgG and IgA antibody levels were dose-dependent in the elderly with significant improvements at 20 and 60 μg respectively. In the young, IgM and IgA were dependent on antigen dose, with a significant improvement at a 60 μg dose. At a 20 μg dose, IgG and IgM levels were comparable between the age groups, whereas IgA levels were significantly higher in the elderly. By contrast, HI antibody titres to the A/Taiwan/1/86 were not dose-dependent.

For the A/Taiwan/1/86 strain, a number of elderly did not respond with HI antibody although isotypic antibody levels to the A/Taiwan/1/86 strain increased significantly in these subjects. This observation that HI did not increase after vaccination whereas isotypic antibody levels increased is in agreement with previous data (41)). The hemagglutination induced by the A/Taiwan/1/86 (H1N1) antigen is not always effectively inhibited by antibodies directed against influenza A/Taiwan/1/86 surface glycoproteins. These antibodies bind to the A/Taiwan/1/86 surface glycoproteins in ELISA, but lack activity in the HI assay. It is unclear at present whether these antibodies are specific for hemagglutinin or neuraminidase.

A 20 μg dose of subunit influenza vaccine elicited IgG and IgM responses to the A/Sichuan/2/87 (H3N2) and A/Taiwan/1/86 (H1N1) components in elderly nursing home residents that were comparable with the responses in the young subjects (52,53). In addition, the IgA response in the elderly treated with the 20 μg dose was higher than the young treated with the same dose (52,53). The 20 μg dose induced higher levels of antibodies in the elderly as compared to the 10 μg, thus the 20 μg dose may induce a higher level of protection in the elderly.

Other authors reported that the HI antibody response to H1N1 strains (A/Chile/1/83) could be improved by increasing the vaccine dose, whereas only tendencies were observed for H3N2 strains (55,56). Our studies (52,53) demonstrate that IgG and IgA antibody levels to the H1N1 vaccine component can be improved by the use of high-dose vaccines, whereas HI antibody levels were not improved by the use of high-dose vaccines (53). In addition, we also found that HI, IgG and IgA antibody levels to the H3N2 strain can be improved by the use of high-dose vaccines (52).

The results obtained in the dose-response studies suggest that the declined response that was observed in ADL disabled nursing home patients (49) could be overcome by the use of high-dose vaccines. However, the populations in the dose-response (52,53) and health status (49) studies may not have been fully comparable. The subjects participating in the dose response study (52,53) were nursing home residents, who were selected as eligible candidates for participation in the vaccination trial, whereas the subjects studied in the functional disability study (49) were representative for the whole population of the nursing home. It was previously observed that only a few differences occurred in the antibody response to influenza vaccine between optimal healthy SENIEUR elderly and nursing home residents, who were selected as eligible candidates for participation in a vaccination study (unpublished results). Thus the benefits of high-dose vaccines in elderly nursing home patients with functional disabilities require further investigation.

Since zinc levels decline with age, a suboptimal zinc status may cause a declined immune capacity; therefore the beneficial effects of zinc supplementation on the antibody response were investigated (57). Antibody levels to the vaccine strains and two related field strains were determined by hemagglutination inhibition. Plasma zinc levels were significantly higher in the zinc supplementation group. However, supplementary zinc had no beneficial effects on the antibody formation to influenza vaccine, which is probably due to the fact that very few subjects were zinc deficient (57). The subjects in this study were independently living elderly and it is possible that zinc deficiencies occur more often in elderly nursing home residents or patients on geriatric wards.

5. The influence of annually repeated vaccinations

There have been conflicting observations about the protection of annually repeated vaccinees. In the seventies, Hoskins et. al reported that annually vaccinated boarding school boys were less protected during an influenza epidemic than boys who had received their first vaccination in the year of the epidemic. Although we have shown recently that these conclusions could not be substantiated after a re-evaluation of their own data (58), several studies between 1966 and 1997 have shown divergent results. Some reported that annually vaccinated people had similar antibody formation as single vaccinated people, others observed a declined antibody formation in annually vaccinated people as compared to those who received only one vaccination.

We performed a metanalysis of thirteen field trials (measuring laboratory confirmed influenza like illness) and 53 serological trials (measuring hemagglutination inhibiting (HI) antibody production) with a total of 19,823 observations. The field data presented a clear homogeneous picture: all field trials concluded that annually repeated vaccinees were equally as well protected as the single vaccinees. The serological studies showed heterogeneous results. Out of 53 trials, nine trials were in favour of single vaccination, seven were in favour of multiple vaccination and the rest showed no difference between multiple and single vaccination. Metanalysis of the available data showed no evidence that annually repeated vaccination influences field or serological protection against influenza.

The heterogeneity between serological studies has been described earlier (24,59-61). Although the post-vaccination HI titre is a valuable surrogate marker for field protection, it may depend on a number of co-factors which are imperfectly controlled by the study design, among others, pre-vaccination titre, study design and study population characteristics (age *per se*, individual history of previous exposure to natural influenza, especially the effect of original antigenic sin (62), health state, etc.). In an attempt to avoid these biases, we conducted a longitudinal study in healthy elderly and young volunteers (screened with the SENIEUR protocol (63)), where we vaccinated the volunteers annually with commercially available influenza vaccine. We measured the HI antibody response (42) and ELISA antibodies (43) during three years. Both methods showed no decrease of antibody levels to the influenza vaccination strains after annually repeated vaccination in healthy elderly and young persons. More importantly, the HI antibody response to the influenza B strains in the vaccine improved in the elderly after annually repeated vaccination, reaching the same level as the young persons after the second vaccination. The IgG antibody levels, measured by ELISA, increased after annually repeated vaccination in young and elderly subjects, whereas the IgA levels were found to decrease slightly in both age groups.

These data support the advice to vaccinate (elderly) people at risk for serious morbidity and mortality by influenza every year. More so, because we found that annually repeated vaccination results in a higher amount of antibodies present during the year after vaccination (43). The level of these remaining antibodies increased progressively with increasing number of vaccinations. The amount of antibodies that is formed after vaccination is related to the protection against influenza (64,65). If by annually repeated vaccination this amount increases, protection will also increase.

By applying different methods to estimate the protection afforded by annually repeated vaccination (metanalysis of published data and antibody measurement with two different assays) the unanimous conclusion is that annually repeated vaccination does not result in lower protection (directly measured by morbidity and mortality) or in lower antibody levels (indirect protection measure) in elderly and young persons.

6. The effect of annually repeated vaccination on antibody quality

The quality of the antibody response can be measured *in vitro* by several methods. The avidity of antibodies, also referred to as the average affinity, is used to describe the binding strength of a population of polyclonal antibodies with a polyvalent antigen. The maturation of antibodies during repeated exposure to specific epitopes results in high affinity antibodies that are qualitatively better in binding to the specific epitope. After repeated vaccination with influenza virus one can therefore expect to find an increase of affinity, or avidity. The avidity of antibodies can be measured with an ELISA method using chaotropic agents like urea or sodium-thiocyanate (66-70).

Little is known about the avidity maturation of antibodies in the ageing process. Some studies suggest a decline with age (66,71), but the consequence of ageing of the immune system for the antibody avidity to influenza antigens is not yet clear. The avidity of IgG and IgA antibodies was measured in the elderly and young persons who participated in the longitudinal study on the effect of annually repeated vaccination on the antibody response (43). The avidity was measured to two vaccine strains: A/Taiwan/1/86 (H1N1) and A/Beijing/353/89 (H3N2). IgG and IgA antibodies had increasing avidities to both vaccine strains after annually repeated vaccination, although more prominent in the young than in the elderly persons.

The quality of the immune response can also be expressed as the neutralising capacity of antibodies. In the cohorts of annually vaccinated elderly and young persons who participated in the longitudinal influenza study, the neutralising capacity of antibodies against the A/Taiwan/1/86 (H1N1) vaccine strain was measured with an *in vitro* micro-cytotoxicity test (72). As we have seen for the quantity and avidity of antibodies, annually repeated vaccination results in an increase of neutralising antibodies. It is not so much that these parameters reach higher and higher levels after every subsequent vaccination, but that the level that can still be measured one year after vaccination increases from year to year. This higher overall level of neutralising antibodies results in better protection. Unfortunately, the height of the neutralising antibody titre was only correlated to the amount of IgG and IgA antibody in the serum and not with the avidity of the antibodies. In other words, the neutralising capacity as measured by the *in vitro* micro-cytotoxicity assay is not related to the *in vitro* avidity of the antibodies. This may be caused by the fact that the *in vitro* avidity index is merely a measure of the overall binding activity of a broad spectrum of antibody specificities, not necessarily having specific neutralising capacity in the micro-cytotoxicity assay.

7. In conclusion

In healthy elderly people antibody production capacity following influenza vaccination is retained. The antibody response to some strains is lower in the elderly, but this is probably related to differences in previous exposures.

Elderly people with a poor health status, as determined by the ADL-scale, have lower antibody responses following influenza vaccination. However, they still have a significant improvement in antibody titres following vaccination. Therefore it can be assumed that the protection to influenza infection will also be increased.

In elderly people, the antibody response following influenza vaccination can be improved by increasing the vaccine dose.

Annually repeated influenza vaccinations do not lead to lower antibody responses in elderly people. Moreover our data present evidence that annually repeated influenza vaccination reinforces immunity to influenza.

References

[1] Katz RS. Influenza 1918-1919: A study in mortality. Bull.Hist.Med. 1974;48:416-22.

[2] Houseworth J, Langmuir AD. Excess mortality from epidemic influenza, 1957-1966. Am.J.Epidemiol. 1974;100:40-8.

[3] Sprenger MJW, van Naelten MAMG, Mulder PGH, Masurel N. Influenza Mortality and Excess Deaths in the Elderly, 1967-1982. Epidem.Inf. 1989;103:633-41.

[4] Sprenger MJW, Mulder PGH, Beyer WEPh, van Strik R, Masurel N. Impact of influenza on mortality in relation to age and underlying disease, 1967-1989. Int.J.Epidem. 1993;22:334-40.

[5] Couch RB, Kasel JA, Glezen WP, Cate TR, Six HR, Taber LH, Frank AL, Greenberg SB, Zahradnik JM, Keitel WA. Influenza: Its control in persons and populations. J.Infect.Dis. 1986;153:431-40.

[6] Glezen WP. Serious Morbidity and Mortality Associated with Influenza Epidemics. Epidem.Rev. 1993;4:25-44.

[7] Lui K-J, Kendal AP. Impact of influenza epidemics on mortality in the United States from October 1972 to May 1985. Am.J.Public Health 1987;77:712-6.

[8] Barker WH, Mullooly JP. Influenza Vaccination of Elderly Persons: Reduction in Pneumonia an Influenza Hospitalizations and Deaths. JAMA 1980;244:2547-9.

[9] Barker WH, Mullooly JP. Impact of Epidemic Type A Influenza in a Defined Adult Population. Am.J.Epidemiol. 1980;112:798-813.

[10] Barker WH, Mullooly JP. Pneumonia and influenza deaths during epidemics: Implications for prevention. Arch.Intern.Med. 1982;142:85-9.

[11] Mäkelä PH, Jokinen C, Pyhälä R, Mäkelä M, Ruutu P. Use of vaccines for respiratory infections: Strategies for influenza and pneumococcal vaccines. Scand.J.Inf.Dis,suppl. 1990;70:141-8.

[12] Tillett HE, Smith JW, Gooch CD. Excess deaths attributable to influenza in England and Wales: age at death and certified cause. Int.J.Epidemiol. 1983;12:344-52.

[13] Glezen WP, Six HR, Frank AL, et al. Kendal AP, Patriarca PA, editors.Options for the control of influenza. New York: Allan Liss; 1986;Impact of epidemics upon communities and families. p. 63-73.

[14] Centraal Bureau voor de Statistiek. 's Gravenhage: SDU Uitgeverij; 1989;Bevolkingsprognose voor nederland 1988-2050.

[15] Davies JR, Grilli EA, Smith AJ. Infection with influenza A H1N1. 2. The effect of past experience on natural challenge. J.Hyg.Camb. 1986;96:345-52.

[16] Davies JR, Grilli EA, Smith AJ. Influenza A: Infection and reinfection. J.Hyg.Camb. 1984;92:125-7.

[17] Stange KC, Little DW, Blatnik B. Adverse reactions to amantadine prophylaxis of influenza in a retirement home. J.Am.Geriatr.Soc. 1991;39:700-5.

[18] Degelau J, Somani S, Cooper SL, Irvine PW. Occurence of adverse effects and high amantadine concentrations with influenza prophylaxis in the nursing home. J.Am.Geriatr.Soc. 1990;38:428-32.

[19] Degelau J, Somani SK, Cooper SL, Guay DRP, Crossley KB. Amantadine-resistant influenza A in a nursing facility. Arch.Intern.Med. 1992;152:390-2.

[20] Mast EE, Harmon MW, Gravenstein S, Ping Wu S, Arden NH, Circo R, Tyszka G, Kendal AP, Davis JP. Emergence and possible transmission of amantadine-resistant viruses during nursing home outbreaks of influenza A (H3N2). Am.J.Epidemiol. 1991;134:988-97.

[21] Monto AS, Arden NH. Implications of viral resistance to amantadine in control of influenza A. Clin.Infect.Dis. 1992;15:362-7.

[22] Hayden FG, Belshe RB, Clover RD, Hay AJ, Oakes MG, Soo W. Emergence and apparent transmission of Rimantadine-resistant influenza A virus in families. N.Engl.J.Med. 1989;321:1696-702.

[23] Corfield T. Tailor made sialidase inhibitors home in on influenza virus. Glycobiology 1993;3:413-5.

[24] Beyer WEPh, Palache AM, Baljet M, Masurel N. Antibody induction by influenza vaccines in the elderly: a review of the literature. Vaccine 1989;7:385-94.

[25] Patriarca PA, Weber JA, Parker RA, Hall WN, Kendal AP, Bregman DJ, Schonberger LB. Efficacy of influenza vaccine in nursing homes: Reduction in illness and complications during an influenza A (H3N2) epidemic. JAMA 1985;253:1136-9.

[26] Meiklejohn G, Hall H. Unusual outbreak of influenza A in a Wyoming nursing home. J.Am.Geriatr.Soc. 1987;35:742-6.

[27] Barker WH, Raubertas R, Menegus M, et al. Hannoun C, Kendal AP, Klenk HD, Ruben FL, editors.Options for the control of influenza II. Amsterdam: Elsevier Science Publishers b.v.; 1993;Case control study of influenza vaccine effectiveness in preventing pneumonia hospitalization among older persons, Monroe County, New York, 1989-1992. p. 143-51.

[28] Monto AS, Ohmit SE, Foster DA, et al. Hannoun C, Kendal AP, Klenk HD, Ruben FL, editors.Options for the control of influenza II. Amsterdam: Elsevier Science Publishers B.V.; 1993;Case-control study in Michigan on prevention of hospitalization by vaccination, 1989-1991. p. 135-41.

[29] Nichol KL, Margolis KL, Wuorenma J, Von Sternberg TL. The efficacy and cost effectiveness of vaccination against influenza among elderly persons living in the community. N.Engl.J.Med. 1994;331:778-84.

[30] Govaert ThME, Thijs CTMCN, Masurel N, Sprenger MJW, Dinant GJ, Knottnerus JA. The efficacy of influenza vaccination in elderly individuals: A randomized double-blind placebo-controlled trial. JAMA 1994;272(21):1661-5.

[31] Govaert ThME, Thijs CTMCN, Masurel N, Sprenger MJW, Dinant GJ, Knottnerus JA. De effectiviteit van influenzavaccinatie bij ouderen; een gerandomiseerd, dubbelblind, placebo-gecontroleerd onderzoek. Ned.Tijdschr.Geneesk. 1995;139(42):2140-3.

[32] Gross PA, Hermogenes AW, Sacks HS, Lau J, Levandowski RA. The efficacy of influenza vaccine in elderly persons. A meta- analysis and review of the literature. Ann.Intern.Med. 1995;123(7):518-27.

[33] Nicholson KG, Baker DJ, Chakraverty P, Farquhar A, Hurd D, Kent J, Litton PA, Smith SH. Immunogenicity of inactivated influenza vaccine in residential homes for elderly people. Age and Ageing 1992;21:182-8.

[34] Mostow SR, Schoenbaum SC, Dowdle WR, Coleman MT, Kaye HS. Studies with inactivated influenza vaccines purified by zonal centrifugation. 1. Adverse reactions and serological responses. Bull.World Health Organ. 1969;41:525-30.

[35] Phair J, Kauffman CA, Bjornson A, Adams L, Linnemann C. Failure to respond to influenza vaccine in the aged: correlation with B-cell number and function. J.Lab.Clin.Med. 1978;92:822-8.

[36] Feery BJ, Evered MG, Morrison EM. Different protection rates in various groups of volunteers given subunit influenza virus vacine in 1976. J.Infect.Dis. 1979;139:237-41.

[37] Strassburg MA, Greenland S, Sorvillo FJ, Lieb LE, Habel LA. Influenza in the elderly: report of an outbreak and review of vaccine effectiviness reports. Vaccine 1986;4:38-44.

[38] Coles FB, Balzano GJ, Morse DL. An outbreak of influenza A (H3N2) in a well immunized nursing home population. J.Am.Geriatr.Soc. 1992;40:589-92.

[39] D'Alesio DJ, Cox PM, Dick EC. Failure of inactivated influenza vaccine to protect an aged population. JAMA 1969;210:485-9.

[40] Hoskins TW, Davies JR, Smith AJ, Miller CL, Allchin A. Assessment of Inactivated Influenza-A Vaccine After Three Outbreaks of Influenza-A at Christs's Hospital. The Lancet 1979;i,33-5.

[41] Remarque EJ, de B, I, Boersma WJ, Masurel N, Ligthart GJ. Altered antibody response to influenza H1N1 vaccine in healthy elderly people as determined by HI, ELISA, and neutralization assay. J Med Virol 1998;55(1):82-7.

[42] de Bruijn IA, Remarque EJ, Beyer WEPh, LeCessie S, Masurel N, Ligthart GJ. Annually repeated influenza vaccination improves humoral responses to several influenza virus strains in healthy elderly. Vaccine 1997;15(12/13):1323-9.

[43] de Bruijn IA, Remarque EJ, Jol-van der Zijde CM, van Tol MJD, Westendorp RGJ, Knook DL. Quality and quantity of the humoral immune response in healthy elderly and young subjects after annually repeated influenza vaccination. J.Infect.Dis. 1999;179(1):31-6.

[44] Pyhälä R, Kinnunen L, Kumpulainen V, Ikonen N, Kleemola M, Cantell K. Vaccination-induced HI antibody to influenza A(H1N1) viruses in poorly primed adults under circumstances of low antigenic drift. Vaccine 1993;11:1013-7.

[45] McElhaney JE, Meneilly GS, Lechelt KE, Beattie BL, Bleackley RC. Antibody response to whole-virus and split-virus influenza vaccines in successful ageing. Vaccine 1993;11:1055-60.

[46] Powers DC, Belshe RB. Effect of age on cytotoxic T lymphocyte memory as well as serum and local antibody responses elicited by inactivated influenza virus vaccine. J.Infect.Dis. 1993;167:584-92.

[47] Remarque EJ, Nijhuis EWP, Hinloopen B, Nagelkerken L, van der Velde EA, and Ligthart GJ. Correlation between the antibody response to influenza vaccine and helper T cell subsets in healthy ageing. Vaccine 1996;14(2):127-30.

[48] Nijhuis EWP, Remarque EJ, Hinloopen B, Van der Pauw-Kraan T, Van Lier RAW, Ligthart GJ, Nagelkerken L. Age-Related increase in the fraction of $CD27^{-}CD4^{+}$ T cells and IL-4 production as a feature of $CD4^{+}$ T cell differentiation *in vivo*. Clin.Exp.Immunol. 1994;96:528-34.

[49] Remarque EJ, Cools HJM, Boere TJ, van der Klis RJ, Masurel N, and Ligthart GJ. Functional disability and antibody response to influenza vaccine in elderly patients in a Dutch nursing home. Br.Med.J. 1996;312(20 April):1015.

[50] Gross PA, Quinnan GV, Weksler ME, Setia U, Douglas RG. Relation of chronic disease and immune response to influenza vaccine in the elderly. Vaccine 1989;7:303-8.

[51] de Greef GE, van Tol MJD, Kallenberg CGM, van Staalduinen GJ, Remarque EJ, Tjandra YI, Hijmans W. Influence of ageing on antibody formation in vivo after immunisation with the primary T-cell dependent antigen *Helix pomatia* haemocyanin. Mech.Ageing Dev. 1992;66:15-27.

[52] Remarque EJ, van Beek WCA, Ligthart GJ, Borst RJA, Nagelkerken L, Palache AM, Sprenger MJW, Masurel N. Improvement of the Immunoglobulin Subclass Response to Influenza Vaccine in Elderly Nursing-Home Residents by the use of High-Dose Vaccines. Vaccine 1993;11:649-54.

[53] Remarque EJ, de Jong JMA, Masurel N, Ligthart GJ. Dose-dependent antibody response to influenza H1N1 vaccine component in elderly nursing home residents. .Exp.Gerontol. 1999; in press.

[54] Powers DC. Effect of age on serum immunoglobulin G subclass antibody responses to inactivated influenza virus vaccine. J.Med.Virol. 1994;43:57-61.

[55] Gross PA, Quinnan GV, Weksler ME, Gaerlan PF, Denning CR. Immunization of elderly people with high doses of influenza vaccine. J.Am.Geriatr.Soc. 1988;36:209-12.

[56] Sullivan KM, Monto AS, Foster DA. Antibody response to inactivated influenza vaccines of various antigenic concentrations. J.Infect.Dis. 1990;161:333-5.

[57] Remarque EJ, Witkamp L, Masurel N, Ligthart GJ. Zinc supplementation does not enhance antibody formation to influenza virus vaccine in the elderly. Aging Immunol.Infect.Dis. 1993;4:17-23.

[58] Beyer WEPh, de Bruijn IA, Palache AM, Westendorp RGJ, Osterhaus ADME. The plea against annual influenza vaccination? "The Hoskins' Paradox" revisited. Vaccine 1997;

[59] Palache AM, Beyer WEPh, Sprenger MJW, Masurel N, De Jonge S, Vardy A, Charpentier B, Noury J, van Beek WCA, Borst RJA, et al. Antibody response after influenza immunization with various vaccine doses: A double-blind, placebo-controlled, multi- centre, dose-response study in elderly nursing-home residents and young volunteers. Vaccine 1993;11:3-9.

[60] Palache AM, Beyer WEPh, Lüchters G, Völker R, Sprenger MJW, Masurel N. Influenza vaccines: The effect of vaccine dose on antibody response in primed populations during the ongoing interpandemic period. A review of the literature. Vaccine 1993;11:892-908.

[61] Beyer WEPh, Palache AM, Sprenger MJW, Hendriksen E, Tukker JJ, Darioli R, van der Water GL, Masurel N, Osterhaus ADME. Effects of repeated annual influenza vaccination on vaccine sero-response in young and elderly adults. Vaccine 1997;14(14):1331-40.

[62] Webster RG, Kasel JA, Couch RB, Laver WG. Influenza subunit vaccines II. Immunogenicity and original antigenic sin in humans. J.Infect.Dis. 1976;134:48-58.

[63] Ligthart GJ, Corberand JX, Geertzen HGM, Meinders AE, Knook DL, Hijmans W. Necessity of the assessment of health status in human immunogerontological studies: evaluation of the SENIEUR protocol. Mech.Ageing Dev. 1990;55:89-105.

[64] Potter CW, Oxford JS. Determinants of immunity to influenza in man. Br.Med.Bull. 1979;35:69-75.

[65] Wesselius-de Casparis A, Masurel N, Kerrebijn KF. Field trial with human and equine influenza vaccines in children; protection and antibody titres. Bull.World Health Organ. 1972;46:151

[66] Schoub BD, Blackburn NK, Johnson S, McAnerney JM, Miller B. Low antibody avidity in elderly chickenpox patients. J.Med.Virol. 1992;37:113-5.

[67] Konradsen HB. Quantity and avidity of pneumococcal antibodies before and up to five years after pneumococcal vaccination of elderly persons. Clin.Infect.Dis. 1995;22(1):616-20.

[68] Brokstad KA, Cox RJ, Major D, Wood JM, Haaheim LR. Cross-reaction but no avidity change of the serum antibody response after influenza vaccination. Vaccine 1995;13(16):1522-8.

[69] Ward KN, Dhaliwal W, Ashworth KL, Clutterbuck EJ, Teo CG. Measurement of antibody avidity for hepatitis C Virus distinguishes primary antibody responses from passively acquired antibody. J.Med.Virol. 1994;43:367-72.

[70] Pullen GR, Fitzgerald MG, Hosking CS. Antibody avidity determination by ELISA using thiocyanate elution. J.Immunol.Methods 1986;86(1):83-7.

[71] Kishimoto S, Takahama T, Mizumachi H. In vitro immune response to the 2,4,6-TNP determinant in aged C57BL/6J mice: Changes in the humoral immune response, avidity for the TNP determinant and responsiveness to LPS effect with aging. J.Immunol. 1976;116:294-300.

[72] de Bruijn IA, van der Klis RJ, Remarque EJ, Westendorp RGJ, Knook DL. Neutralizing capacity of antibodies after annually repeated influenza vaccination in elderly and young individuals. Submitted 1999

EUCAMBIS: Immunology and Ageing in Europe
G. Pawelec (Ed.)
IOS Press, 2000

Acute Rejection: The Impact of Recipient Age

Benjamin A BRADLEY
University of Bristol Division of Transplantation Sciences
Building 11 Zone A
Southmead Health Services
Westbury on Trym
Bristol BS10 5NB, UK

Abstract:

Do older recipients of clinical transplants have a lower risk of acute rejection? In kidney transplant data analyses this effect is often obscured by inappropriate biostatistical modelling. Mortality attributable to infection, cardiovascular and technical failures needs to be censured from the analysis before the true relationship is revealed. Biopsy-proven episodes of acute rejection are seldom recorded and surrogate outcome measures have to be substituted. A well validated database of 7,250 first cadaveric kidney transplants performed in the United Kingdom and Republic of Ireland between 1985 and 1993 was explored. Recipients whose grafts failed during the first post-transplant week were censured as were any recipients who died with a functioning transplant. Multifactorial analysis identified major factors affecting graft survival in the first year post-transplant. After correction for these major factors increasing recipient age was shown to be associated with decreasing risk of graft failure. Liver transplants in adult recipients over the age of 60 have also been shown to be affected less by acute cellular rejection than in recipients under the age of 60 years at transplant. Corneal transplantation offers a more informative clinical model since grafts are performed across a wider age spectrum. Acute rejection can be directly visualised and accurately recorded by the clinician. Using multifactorial methods 3,213 corneal transplants performed in the United Kingdom and Republic of Ireland between 1987 and 1991 were analysed. After correction for major factors affecting outcome a clear correlation between increasing recipient age and decreasing risk of acute rejection and graft failure were demonstrated. Several known mechanisms might be invoked to account for this phenomenon, namely, replicative senescence, a shrinking T-cell repertoire due to thymic involution, the possible emergence of cross-reactive suppressor T-cell clones and increased susceptibility to immunosuppressive drugs. Is it possible that older recipients of organ transplants are being treated with inappropriate levels of immunosuppression and as a consequence suffering more lethal side effects? This question cannot readily be addressed in the absence of an in-vitro model of acute rejection allowing susceptibility to immunosuppressive drugs to be compared at different ages.

1. GENERAL INTRODUCTION

In theory, transplants beget immortality; in reality older patients suffer more complications and clinicians tend to favour younger recipients. Consequently, when organ supply is restricted as with hearts, elderly recipients have lower priority. This tendency is given credence by the observation that failures are higher in older than in younger patients, but more discerning analyses reveal that the causes of graft failure change with increasing age. Failures due to 'non-immunological causes' increase whilst those due to 'immunological' causes decrease [1,2]. By contrast corneal transplantation (penetrating keratoplasty) is offered to patients of all ages [3] and is a better model for studying age associated changes in acute rejection.

Statistical analysis of risk factors associated with transplants needs to relate to defined clinical outcome measures to ensure observations are interpreted within a rational biological framework. For example, to investigate the impact of age-linked changes in cellular immunity on transplant rejection, the first step would be to look for an association between recipient age and probability of acute rejection. Unfortunately, the definition of acute rejection is based on subjective as well as objective clinical criteria. It varies in severity and differs according to the type of graft. Acute rejection is often reversible with immunosuppressive drugs but recurrences may arise. Some episodes fail to respond and proceed inexorably to drug resistant graft failure which is the major cause of graft loss in the first year. Since reliable data on episodes of acute rejection is often poorly documented, graft failure may be used as a surrogate indicator of outcome.

Graft failure results not only from acute rejection but also other causes including technical failure and 'chronic rejection'. Chronic rejection is a separate pathological process resulting in smooth muscle proliferation, intimal thickening, obliteration of vascular lumina and ischaemia. After transplantation technical failures tend to occur during the first week and chronic rejection becomes increasingly prevalent after the first year. Cardiovascular disease and other complications leading to 'death with a functioning transplant' occur increasingly with age. Such cases should be identified and censured if the analyses are focussed on age associated changes in immune responses [2]. With these caveats the analysis of clinical transplant databases offer an effective tool for investigating the impact of age on acute rejection.

Much is known of the age-linked restructuring of T-cell immunity [4] and several mechanisms might be invoked to explain the observed decline in acute rejection. One practical benefit of understanding these mechanisms might be to use lower doses of immunosuppressive drugs in older transplant recipients, but this requires a better understanding of the relationship between drug efficacy and age. A wider knowledge of underlying immunological mechanisms may also lead to substantial improvements in long term graft survival, allowing clinicians to extend the age range of patients benefiting from these vital procedures.

In this chapter the available clinical data is summarised with a view to planning future investigations into mechanisms.

2. KIDNEY TRANSPLANTS

The phenomenon of age associated decline in acute rejection in kidney transplantation has been largely obscured by inappropriate statistical analyses [2]. The prevailing experience amongst clinicians is that kidney transplantation is associated with more life threatening complications such as cardio-vascular disease, infection and cancer in the elderly compared to younger patients. Most complications in older recipients might be avoided by better patient selection and modifications in immunosuppressive drug therapy. Pharmacokinetic studies of these drugs reveal little difference in metabolism and bio-availability with age [5]. However, studies addressing changes in drug efficacy specifically in the context of T-cell mediated allo-immunity, a mechanism central to acute rejection, have not yet been done. Biopsies of acutely rejecting kidney grafts show destruction of the architecture and heavy infiltration with T-cells. Few multi-centre databases record *biopsy-proven* acute rejection episodes, hence analyses of acute rejection have to rely on surrogate outcome measures, such as raised creatinine levels, return to dialysis, treatment with anti-rejection therapy (e.g. OKT3, ATG or bolus prednisolone) and graft failure. The major cause of graft failure during the first post-transplant year is acute rejection resistant to anti-rejection therapy.

A simple retrospective analysis was conducted on 7,250 first cadaveric transplants performed between 1985 and 1993 in 27 centres in the United Kingdom and Republic of Ireland. The accuracy of graft failure as a surrogate for acute rejection was improved by censuring failures within the first seven days and after the first year.

Early failures were assumed to result from surgical complications and late failure beyond one year was assumed to be caused increasingly by chronic rejection and recurrent disease. Cases of 'death with a functioning transplant' were censured from the analysis for the reasons already stated.

Graft failure was influenced by multiple factors and the relative risk (RR) associated with each was evaluated using Cox's proportional hazards regression model. These methods and their application have been described in detail elsewhere [6,7]. The influence of a particular factor on outcome, in this case the probability of graft failure within the first post-transplant year, was expressed as a 'relative risk' (RR). Each factor was stratified into two or more levels and one of these was chosen as a reference or baseline and given an RR of 1.00. Table 1 gives the RRs associated with the major factors affecting graft survival within the first year.

Table 1. Multifactorial analysis of first cadaveric kidney transplants in the United Kingdom and Republic of Ireland performed between 1985 and 1993. *Outcome measure: relative risk of graft failure between 8-365 days post-transplant.*

Factor	Level (baseline)	RR	95% CI	P-value
Year of transplant	(1985-87)	(1.00)		
	1988-90	0.73	0.58-0.91	0.01
	1991-93	0.63	0.54-0.86	<0.00
Sex match	(other)	(1.00)		
	female to male	0.78	0.63-0.97	0.03
Donor age	0-18	1.28	0.99-1.67	0.07
	(19-55)	(1.00)		
	56+	1.86	1.48-2.33	<0.00
Donor cause of death	(trauma)	(1.00)		
	non-trauma	1.43	1.16-1.87	<0.00
Donor kidney	(left)	(1.00)		
	Right	0.92	0.76-1.11	0.39
HLA matching	(beneficial)	(1.00)		
	non-beneficial	1.44	1.11-1.87	0.01
Shipping	(local)	(1.00)		
	Exported	1.17	0.94-1.45	0.16
Recipient age at transplant	0-9	2.32	1.27-4.25	0.01
	10-19	1.33	0.90-1.98	0.15
	20-29	1.42	1.06-1.90	0.03
	30-39	1.22	0.91-1.64	0.19
	40-49	1.08	0.81-1.42	0.61
	(50-59)	(1.00)		
	60+	1.40	1.02-1.92	0.04

RR = relative risk. **95% CI** = 95% confidence interval of RR. **P-value** = probability of relative risk differing from baseline (1.00) by chance.

The major factors adversely associated with an increased probability of graft failure during the post-transplant interval between 8 and 365 days were:

- the year during which the graft was performed. These differences reflected overall improvements in therapeutic procedures. Thus the 1991-93 era was associated with a lower RR indicating better graft survival than the 1985-87 era.
- sex mis-matching as illustrated by female to male transplants having a lower RR than all other gender combinations. This phenomenon could be attributed in part to mismatching for the male associated histocompatibility antigen, H-Y.
- kidneys from donors aged 19-55 years appeared optimal, but below and above this age RR was increased. This may have been due to small size and age associated decline in renal function, respectively.
- kidneys from donors dying from non-traumatic causes were associated with higher RR than donors dying from traumatic causes. This may have reflected the influence of different intensive care regimens on the donor's kidney.
- HLA mis-matching was important. Beneficial matching, defined as a mismatch for no more than one allele at the HLA-A and B loci combined together with zero mismatches for HLA-DR alleles, was superior to non-beneficial matching.
- organs shipped between centres had a higher RR than those used local to the donor's centre. Shipped organs may have suffered from two effects; a tendency for retrieving centres to export donor kidneys of lesser quality and the cumulative effect of cold ischaemia on shipped kidneys
- and the recipient's age at transplant (Figure 1).

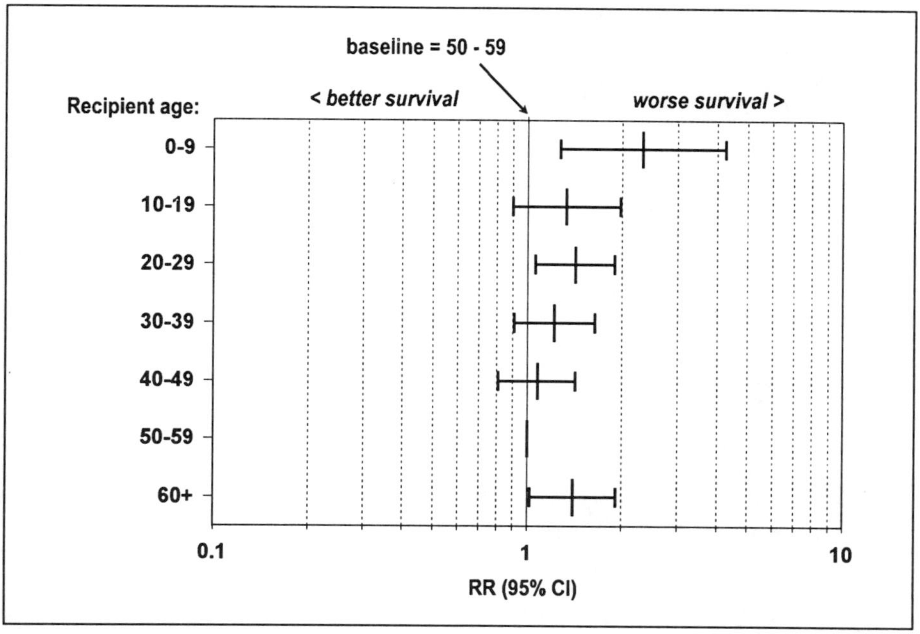

Figure 1. Recipient age in years at the time of kidney transplant plotted against the relative risk (RR) of graft failure with 95% confidence interval (95% CI). RR is expressed relative to a baseline of 50-59 years. *Outcome measure:RR of graft failure between 8-365 days post-transplant (see text for details)*

The independent effect of age was measured against a baseline of 50-59 years as illustrated in figure 1. A trend towards declining RR with increasing age occurs up to the age of 59 was observed. RR increased in the 60+ age group due to unknown causes. Takemoto and Terasaki showed that the proportion of failures attributed to technical, non-immunological and immunological causes changed with recipient age. Immunological failures peaked at around 30 and declined steadily thereafter, whereas non-immunological causes peaked at 60 [1].

3. LIVER TRANSPLANTATION

Liver transplants are uniquely different from other types of vascularised organ transplant in so far as they are less dependent on HLA matching and suffer less chronic graft vasculopathy or 'chronic rejection'. Nonetheless, as with all transplants they appear to be at risk of being acutely rejected during the first post-transplant year. Zetterman and colleagues recently showed that older recipients of primary liver grafts had significantly less 'acute cellular rejection' as assessed by biopsy, at one year post-transplant than younger recipients [25]. A cohort of liver transplants performed between 1990 and 1994 at several centres in the United States were divided into 600 recipients aged below 60 and 135 aged above 60. Children and those with fulminant hepatic failure were censured from the database. As with kidney transplants mortality at one year due to infections, myocardial infarction, and cerebrovascular disease was significantly higher in the older group but the probability of acute rejection was less.

4. CORNEAL TRANSPLANTATON

Historically, corneal transplantation is the longest established type of transplant; the first successful penetrating keratoplasty was recorded in 1905 [8]. Within the context of these studies corneal transplantation differs from vascularised organs in several important ways. Firstly, corneas can be retrieved from a wide range of non-heart beating donors and sufficient tissue is available to satisfy demand. Secondly, diseases leading to corneal blindness are seldom systemic or life-threatening. Thirdly, corneal transplants require only topical immunosupression leading to fewer treatment related complications. Fourthly, experimental evidence suggests the eye's anterior chamber is an 'immunologically privileged site' evoking weaker immune responses. The lack of vasculature in the corneal bed, the lack of donor dendritic cells in the graft and the high expression of apoptosis-inducing molecules such as Fas (CD95) in the anterior chamber are contributory causes. Nonetheless, corneal transplants evoke T-cell mediated acute rejection, most episodes of which are suppressible with topical steroids. But, as with kidney transplants, drug resistant acute rejection accounts for the majority of graft failure during the first year.

The critical layer of the cornea is the inner mono-layer of cells termed the 'corneal endothelium'. In man corneal endothelial cells are growth-arrested whereas in rabbits and rats they replenish themselves. In man the critical threshold for endothelial cell density is around 2,000 cells per mm^2. Below this density the pumping function of the monolayer is compromised and water which is normally removed from the middle stromal layer of the cornea accumulates leading to oedema, opacification and blindness. Unlike acute rejection in kidney transplants, the process can be directly observed clinically in corneal grafts. Several patterns of rejection are distinguishable. Signs include corneal epithelial and stromal oedema, endothelial folding, keratic precipitates, anterior chamber cells and flare. In 'low risk' recipients the reported incidence is between 2% and 35% but in 'high risk' recipients it increases to 66% within the first four years post-transplant. Acute rejection episodes may be observed as early as two weeks or as long as 15 years after transplantation, but 70% occur within the first year [9].

Briefly the mechanism of acute rejection involves antigen from transplanted corneal tissue being picked up by the patient's Langerhans cells in the anterior chamber or surrounding host tissue. These become activated and pass to the draining lymph node where they transform into mature dendritic cells and present donor allo-peptide to naive host T cells ('indirect pathway' of antigen presentation). Naive T cells develop into activated T cells and return via the vasculature to attack the endothelial monolayer of the graft. Unlike kidney transplants, where the process of donor antigen presentation to naive recipient T-cells is 'kick-started' by donor dendritic cells transferred with the organ ('direct pathway' of antigen presentation), corneal tissue has lost all donor dendritic cells as a result of being subjected to tissue culture prior to transplantation. Consequently the host's immune system is activated only via the 'indirect pathway'.

With a view to identifying major factors influencing corneal transplant outcome a multi-centre study involving 3213 transplants performed by 482 ophthalmologists at 216 centres in the United Kingdom between 1987 and 1991 was completed recently [3]. Grafts were followed up for 450 days and outcome was measured either as graft survival, visual acuity or acute rejection. Multifactorial statistical modelling was undertaken to relate each of these outcomes to graft characteristics. Proportional hazards regression was used for assessing graft survival and time to the first rejection episode. In the case of graft survival and acute rejection results were expressed as RR (Table 2a and c). For visual acuity multiple linear regression was used following $\log_e$ transformation of the calculated product of 'visual acuity'. Thus visual acuity of 6/24 (=0.25) is expressed as $\text{Log}_e\, 0.25 = -1.4$. This was termed the regression coefficient (see footnote table 2b).

Table 2. Multifactorial analysis of corneal transplants in the United Kingdom and Republic of Ireland performed between 1987 and 1991. *a) Outcome measure: relative risk (RR) of graft failure between 0-450 days post-transplant.*

Factor	Level (baseline)	RR	95% CI	P-value
Surgeon experience	(< 50 reports)	(1.00)		
	>50 reports	0.61	0.41-0.91	0.01
Previous grafts	(none)	(1.00)		
	one	1.16	0.73-1.82	0.53
	two	2.59	1.41-4.74	<0.00
	more	2.96	1.40-6.22	<0.00
Reasons for graft	(visual only)	(1.00)		
	visual and other	1.16	0.76-1.76	0.49
	non-visual	1.88	1.1-3.20	0.02
Deep vascularisation	(no)	(1.00)		
	yes	1.53	1.07-2.20	0.02
Stromal oedema	(absent)	(1.00)		
	central	1.39	0.79-2.46	0.25
	diffuse/uniform	1.86	1.15-3.03	0.01
	other	2.85	1.34-6.05	<0.00
Uveal inflammation	(no)	(1.00)		
	Yes	1.78	1.01-3.15	0.05
Suture method	(continuous)	(1.00)		
	Interrupted	1.03	0.72-1.47	0.87
	Mixed	1.57	1.01-2.47	0.05
Recipient age	0-9	4.58	1.76-11.92	<0.00
	10-19	1.85	0.62-5.55	0.27
	20-29	1.50	0.66-3.40	0.33
	30-39	0.86	0.37-2.01	0.73
	40-49	1.13	0.54-2.35	0.76
	50-59	1.00	0.51-1.94	1.00
	60-69	1.19	0.68-2.11	0.54
	70-79	1.20	0.71-2.03	0.50
	(80+)	(1.00)		

95% CI = 95% confidence interval of RR. **P-value** = probability of each level differing from the baseline

Table 2 (continued). Multifactorial analysis of corneal transplants in the United Kingdom and Republic of Ireland performed between 1987 and 1991.*b) Outcome measure: visual acuity(VA) denominator at 12 months post-transplant (i.e. 30 equates to VA of 6/30)*

Factor	Level	Mean	95% CI	P-value
Previous grafts	(none)	(24)		
	one	30	24-37	0.01
	Two	40	26-62	<0.00
	More	40	24-66	0.01
Reasons for graft	(not cosmetic)	(24)		
	Cosmetic	28	24-36	0.20
Diagnosis	(keratoconus)	(24)		
	Primary EF	27	19-37	0.47
	secondary EF	46	33-63	<0.00
	herpes zoster keratosis	35	26-48	<0.00
	other inflammation	37	28-51	<0.00
	stromal dystrophy	24	16-34	0.83
	Trauma	59	40-88	<0.00
	Others	61	43-87	<0.00
Glaucoma	(no)	(24)		
	Yes	46	37-57	<0.00
Pre-op. visual acuity	(<6/60)	(24)		
	<6/24	16	14-19	<0.00
	>6/24	15	12-19	<0.00
	Unrecorded	22	11-46	0.77
Graft size-sum	(<14.5)	(24)		
	<0.25	22	19-26	0.20
	>0.25	20	17-24	0.01
Graft size-difference	(0 mm)	(24)		
	<0.25 mm	21	17-25	0.03
	>0.25mm	22	19-26	0.08
Recipent age	0-9	39	14-109	0.25
	10-19	15	10-23	<0.00
	20-29	18	13-25	0.02
	30-39	16	11-22	<0.00
	40-49	17	12-23	<0.00
	50-59	17	12-23	<0.00
	60-69	18	14-24	<0.00
	70-79	20	16-25	0.02
	(80+)	(24)		

Mean = *mean VA denominator*. (24) = *denominator for baseline VA.* **95% CI** = *95% confidence interval.of mean VA..* **P-value** = *probability of mean VA differing from the baseline value (24) by chance*

Table 2 (continued). Multifactorial analysis of corneal transplants in the United Kingdom and Republic of Ireland performed between 1987 and 1991. *c) Outcome measure: relative risk* **(RR)** *of first acute rejection episode within 0-450 days post-transplant*

Factor	Level (baseline)	RR	95% CI	P-value
Previous grafts in operated eye	(none)	(1.00)		
	one	1.39	0.92-2.11	0.12
	two	2.66	1.56-4.54	<0.00
	more	2.75	1.34-5.65	0.01
Diagnosis	(keratoconus)	(1.00)		
	primary EF	1.48	0.68-3.24	0.32
	secondary EF	2.35	1.17-4.69	0.02
	herpes zoster keratosis	1.99	0.99-3.98	0.05
	other inflammation	2.43	1.21-4.86	0.01
	stromal dystrophy	0.98	0.30-3.20	0.97
	trauma	1.94	0.88-4.30	0.10
	others	2.28	1.09-4.76	0.03
Glaucoma	(no)	(1.00)		
	yes	1.52	1.05-2.21	0.03
Graft size-sum	(<14.5)	(1.00)		
	<0.25	1.43	0.99-2.06	0.06
	>0.25	1.58	1.08-2.31	0.02
Recipient age	0 to 9	4.32	1.43-13.01	<0.01
	10 to 19	2.60	0.99-6.85	0.05
	20 to 29	2.40	1.16-5.00	0.02
	30 to 39	1.93	0.97-3.87	0.06
	40 to 49	1.55	0.78-3.08	0.21
	50 to 59	1.43	0.76-2.71	0.27
	60 to 69	1.32	0.75-2.34	0.34
	70 to 79	1.19	0.70-2.04	0.52
	(80+)	(1.00)		

95% CI = *95% confidence interval of the RR.* **P-value** = *probability of difference between each level of a factor and the baseline (1.00) being attributable to chance.*

3.1. Factors associated with Graft Survival

The major factors adversely influencing graft survival between 0 and 450 days post-transplant were:

- the surgeon's experience as reflected in the number of transplants performed
- previously failed grafts.
- deep vascularisation of the corneal bed prior to surgery as reflected in a higher RR of graft failure. Interestingly, this was not associated with increased RR of acute rejection (see below)
- stromal oedema
- inflammation of the uvea
- RR was higher if mixed interrupted and continuous sutures were used.

and the recipient's age at transplant (Figure 2).

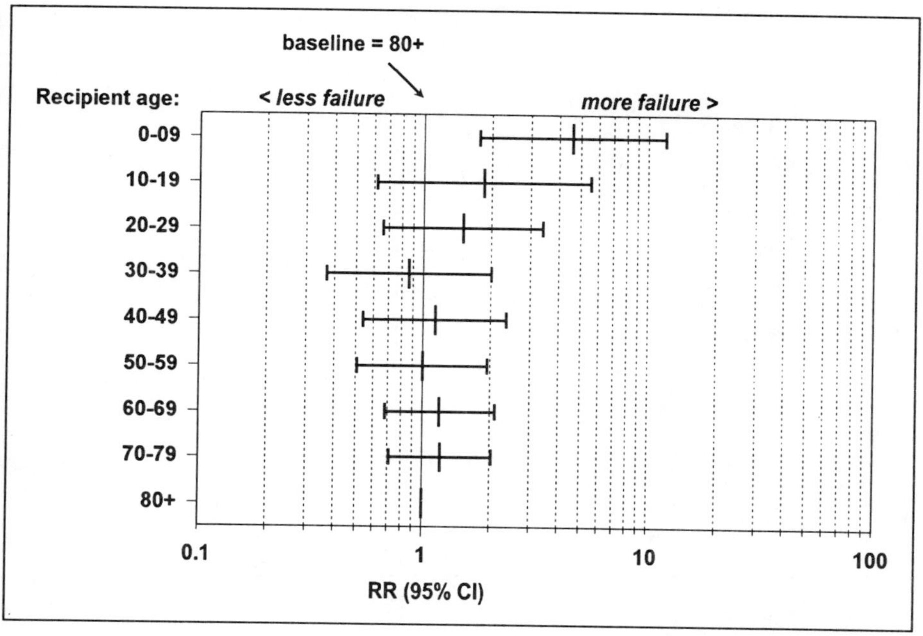

Figure 2. Recipient age in years at the time of corneal transplant plotted against the relative risk (RR) of graft failure with 95% confidence interval (95% CI). RR is expressed against a baseline of 80+ years. *Outcome measure:RR of graft failure between 0-450 days post-transplant (see text for details)*

The independent effect of age is illustrated in figure 2 against a baseline of 80+ years. RR declines progressively with each decade up to 30 years. Above 30 recipient age seems to have no significant impact on graft survival.

3.2. Factors associated with poorer post-transplant visual acuity

The major factors adversely affecting visual acuity were found to be:

- previously failed grafts
- a diagnosis of stromal dystrophy and primary endothelial failure which was associated with a poorer RR than the baseline keratoconus.
- the presence of glaucoma
- poor pre-operative visual acuity
- large grafts which had better visual acuity despite being at greater risk of acute rejection (see below)
- and recipient age at transplant.
-

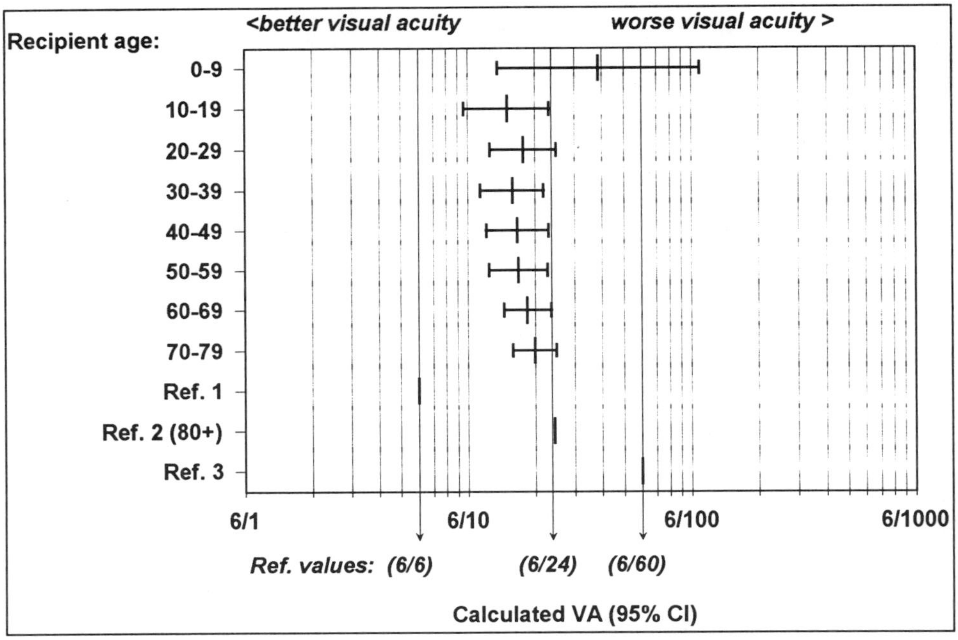

Figure 3. Recipient age in years at the time of corneal transplant plotted against visual acuity at twelve months after grafting with 95% confidence interval (95% CI). *Outcome measure:visual acuity at 12 months post-transplant on a logarithmic scale. The values Ref. 1, 2 and 3 indicate where visual acuities of 6/6, 6/24 and 6/60 would plot (see text for further details).*

The association between age at transplant and visual acuity twelve months post-transplant is illustrated in figure 3. Post-operative visual acuity declines with each decade despite better graft survival and less acute rejection (see below). Declining visual acuity reflects age associated changes in the lens and the retina .

3.3. Factors associated with increased probability of acute rejection

The major factors adversely affecting acute rejection were:

- previously failed grafts
- a diagnosis of secondary endothelial failure and other inflammatory diseases as reflected in a significantly worse RR than other diagnoses.
- glaucoma
- large grafts were associated with higher RR of acute rejection despite being associated with a lower RR of graft failure.
- and recipient age at the time of transplant.

The independent effect of age on acute rejection was measured against a baseline of 80+ years as illustrated in figure 4. A clear trend towards a decreasing RR with each decade up to 80+ was apparent.

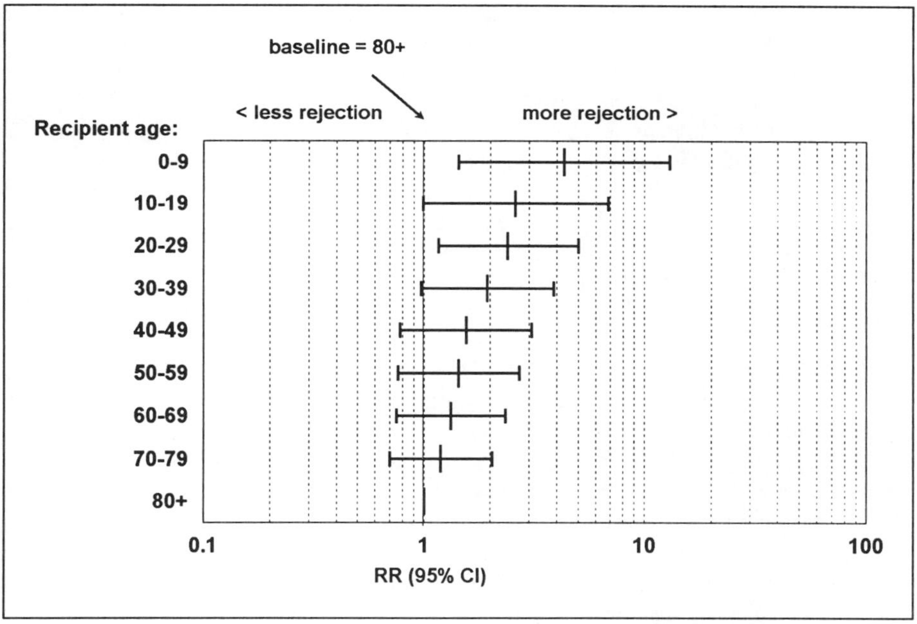

Figure 4. Recipient age in years at the time of corneal transplant plotted against the relative risk (RR) of the first acute rejection episode occuring within 0-450 days post-transplant with 95% confidence interval (95% CI). RR is expressed against a baseline of 80+ years. *Outcome measure: RR of first acute rejection episode between 0-450 days post-transplant (see text for details)*

4. DISCUSSION

The clinical manifestation of acute rejection differs between kidney and corneal transplants, but the underlying process in both involves T cell immunity. Restructuring of T cell immunity occurs with increasing age and the mechanisms underlying this might be responsible for the decline in acute rejection. These mechanisms include, the phenomenon of replicative senescence [10-11], the shrinking T cell repertoire beginning with thymic involution [12], and the expanding population of T-cells with suppresser phenotype [13].

4.1. Replicative senescence

This was first described in 1961 by Hayflick and Moorhead [10]. Today, replicative senescence of cell populations is thought to be determined by the total number of population doublings (i.e. mitoses) a cell has experienced and is reflected in telomere length [11]. T cells from chronically stimulated cultures and peripheral blood lymphocytes from centogenarians both have significantly shortened telomeres compared to younger controls [14]. Shortened telomeres in dividing cells lead to mistakes in replication, and certain genes vital to cell division become inactivated causing arrest in early G1 of the cell cycle. In older transplant recipients clones of allo-reactive memory T cells directed to graft antigens could be compromised according to the number of population doublings experienced since their respective stem cells were established at gestation.

4.2. Thymic involution

Thymic involution begins during the first year after birth and thymic tissue continues to disappear at 3% per year until middle age and 1% thereafter [12]. By extrapolation the thymus would completely disappear by the age of 120! Other lymphoid tissues constituting the non-thymic dependent bulk of spleen and lymph nodes do not involute with age. The net effect on cellular immunity is that the output of post-thymic T cells is dramatically reduced. As an individual gets older cellular immunity relies increasingly on memory T cells. Mice age much faster than man and at 24 months the output of T cells from the thymus is 0.7% of output at birth. The repertoire of clones available to react to newly experienced antigens is more restricted with increasing age as evidenced by a reduction in the range of T cell receptor V-β types. A corollary of this is that the clones of alloreactive cells may simply be absent from the repertoire.

4.3. Cross-reactive suppression

Populations of suppresser T cell clones (CD8+ CD28-) may accumulate throughout life as a result of mucosal challenge with dietary and other foreign peptides. The body's mucosa is continually bombarded by protein in the environment and diet. Allogeneic proteins from other people are transferred through various forms of intimacy. One example was the recent demonstration that kidneys transplanted from relatives who were mismatched for 'non-inherited maternal HLA haplotype' had a significantly higher probability of surviving than those mismatched for the corresponding paternal HLA haplotype [15]. Spousal transplants also appear to have an advantageous survival despite gross HLA mismatching [16]. It is now apparent that mucosally presented peptides are more likely to down-regulate immune responses through the local production of anti-inflammatory cytokines such as Interleukin 4 [17]. Consider how well the gut immune system copes with the continuous barrage of dietary peptides, estimated at 700 tons in an average lifetime! This effect is thought to be mediated by peptide specific T cells that have been polarised to develop along the anti-inflammatory pathway [18].

A significant expansion of the T cell sub-set associated with suppressor cell function, characterised by CD8+ CD28-, occurs with increasing age to the point where they constitute 80% of the CD3+ CD8+ sub-set in healthy centogenerians [13]. Interestingly, this subset is absent from human umbilical cord blood. Cells of this phenotype are known to act on T helper cells to down regulate immune responses [19-21]. Theoretically, many of these peptide specific suppresser T cells may cross-react with allo-specific peptides involved in the initiation of allo-reactive clones [22]. Their influence could be extended through a process of bystander suppression [23] to a degree that would weaken de-novo acute rejection reactions.

4.4. Efficacious immunosupression

Therapeutic levels of immunosuppressive drugs are calculated on the basis of pharmaco-kinetic studies. These change little with age except that young children exhibit 'hyper-alloimmunity' and tend to metabolise the drugs faster than older children or adults [5]. Given that the bulk of T cell tissue decreases with age, and immune deficiency is associated with renal failure and uraemia [24], it is conceivable that an optimal therapeutic effect of these drugs could be achieved in older recipients with doses that would be sub-optimal for younger graft recipients.

4.5. Why investigate the phenomenon?

Exploring the mechanisms underlying this phenomenon is not a wholly academic exercise. There are at least two potential practical applications. Firstly, older transplant recipients are treated with doses of immunosuppressive drugs that are similar to younger recipients and this leads to a much greater risk of life threatening side effects including cardiovascular disease, infections and cancer. Secondly, if mechanisms were better understood they may be exploitable for therapeutic purposes. If for example replicative senescence in donor specific T-cell subsets was shown to be the major cause of decreased acute rejection with age, it might be possible to artificially drive these subsets to exhaustion prior to transplantation. Alternatively, if increased suppresssor subsets accounted for the effect, it may be possible to expand these ex-vivo with a view to modulating rejection. Little progress can be made until an in-vitro model of acute rejection has been developed that truly reflects in-vivo events.

ACNKOWLEDGEMENTS

I wish to thank the staff of the United Kingdom Transplant Support Service, Bristol, UK for providing the analysis of the kidney transplant data. I acknowledge the enormous contribution of the 482 ophthalmic surgeons at 216 centres in the UK and Republic of Ireland who submitted the data. I also wish to acknowledge the following team members of the Corneal Transplant Follow up Study (CTFS) who superbly managed this project over the years and assisted with the analysis: Dr John Armitage, Professor David Easty, Dr Sheila Gore, Dr Chris Rogers and Mr Andy Vail.

REFERENCES

[1] Takemoto S and Terasaki PI. 1988. Donor and recipient age. In Clinical Transplants. P. Terasaki, ed. UCLA Tissue Typing Laboratory, Los Angeles. 345-356.

[2] Tesi RJ, Elkhammas EA, Davies EA et al. 1994. Renal transplantation in older people. The Lancet. 343. 461-464.

[3] Vail A, Gore S, Bradley B A, et al. 1997. Conclusions of the corneal transplant follow up study. Brit. J Ophthalmol. 81. 631-636.

[4] Solano R and Pawalec G. 1998. Molecular and cellular basis of immunosenescence. Mechanisms of ageing and development. 102. 115-129.

[5] Lindholm A and Kahan D. 1993. Influence of cyclosporin pharmacokinetics, trough concentrations and AUC monitoring on outcome after kidney transplantation. Clin. Pharmacol. Ther. 54. 205-218.

[6] Gilks WR, Gore SM and Bradley BA. (1986). Analysing transplant survival data. Transplantation, 42: 46-49.

[7] Gilks WR, Bradley BA, Gore SM. and Selwood NH. (1986). Immunogenetic and clinical factors affecting renal transplantation: a rigorous analysis of data recorded by the UK Transplant Service Transplantation, 42: 39-45.

[8] Zirm E. Eine erfolgreiche totale Keratoplastik. Albrecht von Graefe's archiv fur Ophthalmologie 1906. 64. 580

[9] Bradley B A, Vail A, Gore SM, Rogers CA, Armitage W J, Nicholls SM and Easty DL. Penetrating Keratoplasty in the United kingdom: an interim analysis of the corneal transplant follow up study. In: Clinical Transplants 1993. Eds:Teraski P and Cecka JM. Pub.: UCLA Tissue Typing Laboratory. Chapter 28 293-315

[10] Hayflick L and Moorhead P S. 1961. The serial cultivation of human diploid cell strains. Experimantal Cell Resaerch. 25. 585-621.

[11] Effros RB and Pawelec G. 1997. Replicative senescence of T cells: does the Hayflick Limit lead to immune exhaustion? Immunol. Today. 18. 450-454.

[12] George AJT and Ritter MA. 1996. Thymic involution with ageing: obsolescence or good housekeeping? Immunol. Today 16: 420-425.

[13] Fagnoni FF, Vescovini R, Mazzola M et al. 1996. Expansion of cytotoxic CD8+ CD28- T cells in helathy ageing people, including centenarians. Immunology 88:501-506.

[14] Pawelec G. 1993. Suppressor cells in transplantation immunology: recent advances in T cell immunobiology and cytokine networking contribute to the solution of an old conundrum. Transplant Immunology. 1. 172-182

[15] Burlingham WJ, Grailer AP, Heisey DM, Claas FH, Norman D, Mohanakumar T, Brennan DC, de Fijter H, van Gelder T, Pirsch JD, Sollinger HW, Bean MA. 1998. The effect of tolerance to noninherited maternal HLA antigens on the survival of renal transplants from sibling donors. N Engl J Med. 339:23 1657-64

[16] Terasaki P, Cecka JM, Gjertson DW, and Cho YW. 1997. Spousal and other living renal donor transplants. In: Clinical Transplants 1997. Eds. Ceka JM and Terasaki P. Pub. UCLA Tissue Typing Laboratory, Los Angeles, California. Chapter 25. 269-284.

[17] Ma D, Mellon J and Niederkorn JY. 1997. Oral immunisation as a strategy for enhancing corneal allograft survival. British Journal of Ophthalmology. 81. 778-784.

[18] Bailey M, Hall L, Bland PW and Stokes C. 1994. Production of cytokines by lymphocytes from spleen, mesenteric lymph node and intestinal lamina propria of pigs. Immunology 82. 577-583.

[19] Emara, M. A., and M. F. Mozes. 1995. Cytotoxic T-cell role in renal allograft rejection and regulation. Renal allograft infiltrating cytotoxic T-cell line with suppressor-inducer function. Human Immunology 42:161-166.

[20] Koide J and Engleman EG. 1990. Differences in surface phenotype and mechanism of action between alloantigen-specific CD8+ cytotoxic and suppressor T cell clones. J. Immunol. 144. 32-40.

[21] Ouwehand A J, Baan CC, Roelen DL et al. 1993. The detection of cytotoxic T cells with high-affinity receptors for donor antigens in the transplanted heart as a prognostic factor for graft rejection. Transplantation. 56. 1223-1228.

[22] Mason D. 1998. A very high level of crossreactivity is an essential feature of the T-cell receptor. Immunology Today. 19. 395-404

[23] Vanderlugt CJ and Miller SD. 1996. Epitope spreading. Curr. Opinion in Immunol. 8. 831-836

[24] Chatenoud L, Herbelin A, Beaurain G and Descamps-Latscha B. 1990. Immune deficiency of the uremic patient. Adv. Nephrol. 19:259-266

[25] Zetterman RK, Belle SH, Hoofnagle JH, Lawler S, Wei Y, Everhart F, Wiesner RH, and Lake JR. 1998. Age and liver transplantation. A report of the liver transplant database. Transplantation 66: 500-506

EUCAMBIS: Immunology and Ageing in Europe
G. Pawelec (Ed.)
IOS Press, 2000

T cell differentiation: the side effects of immunological memory

Mike SALMON*[1] & Arne N. AKBAR[#]
**Division of Immunity and Infection, The University of Birmingham. UK*
#Department of Clinical Immunology, The Royal Free Hospital, London. UK

Abstract. During the course of an immune response to antigen, T lymphocyte numbers fluctuate greatly. Initially there is a considerable increase in the number of T cells, which may more than double the total number in the body [1-4]. The extent of this proliferation may be regulated by activation-induced cell death mediated by CD95 (Fas) ligation [5]. At the resolution of infection, the majority of T cells must die by apoptosis, returning T cell numbers to pre-infection levels, or the size of the immune system would have to continually increase [6,7]. These processes are under tight homeostatic control as dysregulation invariably has pathological consequences. The resolution of responses, restoring homeostatic balance, seems to be driven by cytokine deprivation-induced T cell apoptosis [7-9]. However, a fundamental constraint on this process is provided by the requirement for immunological memory. If the immune system is to respond effectively to the same antigen in a more effective manner in future, then some of the cells generated in the primary response must survive. For some years we have investigated the mechanisms and factors that drive the homeostatic control of cell numbers. Some intriguing conclusions can be drawn from this work. As we will attempt to explain: chronic inflammation appears in many respects to be a side effect of the mechanisms that produce and maintain immunological memory.

Rheumatoid arthritis (RA) is a common disease (about 1% of the population world-wide) that is associated with chronic inflammatory damage to synovial joints [10]. For many years, this condition was believed to result from an auto-immune response mediated by "abnormal" T lymphocytes present in the joints. More recently it has become apparent that the synovial T cell population is a normal but highly differentiated population of cells trapped in an environment that actively blocks both their death and emigration. RA provides a clear model to understand the post-thymic differentiation of T cells in humans and the regulation of their numbers.

Immunological abnormalities in rheumatoid arthritis

One of the most intriguing features of rheumatoid arthritis is that it doesn't resolve. During their lifetime most people will suffer from transient events of synovitis or even arthritis, usually associated with infections, but almost invariably these will resolve spontaneously after a short time. In rheumatoid arthritis, the inflammation becomes chronic and persistent. Numerous abnormalities of the rheumatoid immune system were described in trying to address this issue during the 1980's [11]. These could obviously not all be primary genetic peculiarities of the disease for two reasons: firstly, such a large and complex genetic requirement would make RA an extremely rare condition, yet approximately one percent of the population worldwide suffers from this crippling disease. Secondly, many of the "abnormalities" were equally apparent in patients with other chronic inflammatory conditions [12]. This latter observation suggested that the apparent down-regulation of immune responses in chronic inflammation may be a perfectly normal response to excessive stimulation in specific microenvironments.

---

[1] Address correspondence to M.S. at The Division of Immunity and Infection, Rheumatology Group, University of Birmingham, Edgbaston, Birmingham B15 2TT, UK. Email: M.Salmon@bham.ac.uk

A role for T cells in rheumatoid arthritis?

The question of whether T lymphocytes play a significant role in the pathology of rheumatoid arthritis has proved controversial [11,13,14]. Two prominent arguments in favour of a role for T cells in this disease are **1.** the observation that there a quite a lot of them in the inflamed joints of most patients with rheumatoid arthritis [11] and **2.** that the only clearly mapped genetic association with this condition is a class II HLA motif within the third hypervariable region of the DR-β chain. This short stretch of amino acids forms part of the alpha helix bordering the antigen binding cleft [15-17]. As the only known function of class II HLA molecules is to present antigens to $CD4^+$ helper T cells, this strongly supports a role for T cells at some point in the disease process. This amino acid sequence is shared, or highly conserved among HLA alleles that show a positive association with RA, but not those that show no association. Intriguingly, although the association is principally with several subtypes of HLA DR4, a number of completely unrelated molecules that share this sequence also show a strong association with RA. We and others have shown that the association between the conserved HLA motif and RA only holds for patients with severe and persistent disease and also that patients who express two different HLA molecules that both bear the motif do very badly [18-22]. We have previously suggested that this implies a role for class II HLA (and indirectly for T cells) in the switch to persistent and erosive disease [17-19]. However it is equally plausible that the ACR criteria for rheumatoid arthritis do not define a single disease entity [23]. Patients with severe HLA DR-associated RA may actually have a quite separate disease to those who present with mild symptoms. No satisfactory mechanism has been advanced to explain this extremely complex association between the conserved class II HLA motifs and rheumatoid arthritis [17]. On balance it seems that the HLA association does imply a role for T cells in the initiation of RA, but does not really address the issue of chronicity.

T cell populations in rheumatoid joints show a largely polyclonal antigen receptor usage and precursors specific for most T cell recall antigens can be found in this compartment [24-28]; indeed when patients with RA were immunised with influenza vaccine, T cells recognising this antigen were recovered from affected joints within weeks [28]. However, even in experimental lesions induced by a known antigen, the number of cells found within the lesion that actually recognise the causative antigen is very low: between 1:500 and 1:5000 [29,30]. T cell responses are therefore highly specific in their induction, but rapidly lose this specificity by recruitment of unrelated cells to the lesion. In long-standing chronic inflammation, the original causative antigen is likely to remain elusive, and perhaps irrelevant to the persistent process. Having said this, removing T cells was shown many years ago to have a beneficial effect on rheumatoid synovitis [31,32], which does suggest an active role for these cells in the continuing disease process. Antigenically irrelevant cells recruited to the synovium in a non-specific manner but in an activated state may well produce potent levels of inflammatory cytokines for short periods of time, sufficient to drive a macrophage/fibroblast based inflammatory process [11].

T cells removed from rheumatoid synovial tissue or fluid are difficult to stimulate and produce cytokines in very low levels, particularly IL-2 and IFN-γ [11,12,14,33]. These cytokines might have been expected to be prominent in a chronic inflammatory response driven by T cells. Indeed, in the mid 1980's it was argued that this seemingly deficient function of synovial T cells was responsible for the persistence of rheumatoid synovial inflammation, because such a 'defective' response would be unable to resolve spontaneously [11]. In fact, as we will discuss later, this apparent deficiency in T cell responsiveness almost certainly reflects the state of differentiation of synovial T cells.

The progressive differentiation of primed T cells is associated with increasing susceptibility to apoptosis.

Synovial T lymphocytes in RA are almost exclusively antigen-experienced primed cells, expressing the lowest molecular weight isoform of the leukocyte common antigen: CD45RO [34,35]. This results from a well documented preference for migration of primed cells to tissue lesions [34,36]. Until recently no markers were available to distinguish newly primed cells from long established clones. This severely hampered attempts to determine the functional role of T cells in synovial joints. We have described a spectrum of primed $CD4^+$ T cells characterised by an inverse relationship between the expression of two CD45 epitopes: CD45RB and CD45RO [37]. Primed $CD4^+$ T cells progress through many cycles of division from a $CD45RB^{bright}O^{dull}$to a $CD45RB^{dull}O^{bright}$ state (Figure 1). This progressive differentiation defined by the shift from $CD45RB^{bright}$ to $CD45RB^{dull}$ is paralleled by the gradual loss of bcl-2 (an intracellular protein that inhibits apoptosis) and gain of Fas (CD95) expression. Fas is a surface receptor for specific signals that induce apoptosis; consequently these two features are associated with an increased propensity for apoptosis. At the same time,

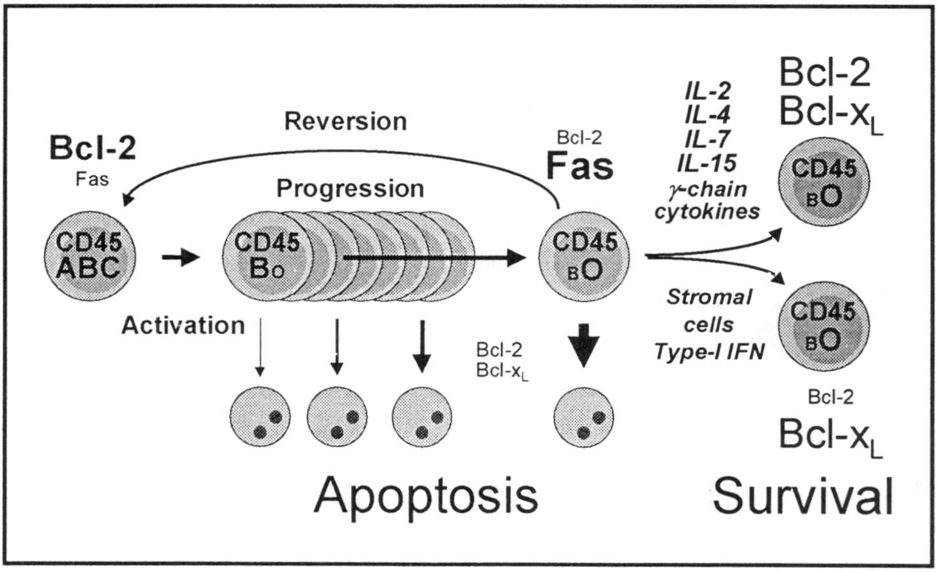

Figure 1. The progressive differentiation of primed T cells is associated with increasing susceptibility to apoptosis. When T cells are recruited from the naïve population, the lose expression of CD45RA, but expression of CD45RB diminishes only slowly with multiple rounds of activation. This progressive change in primed T cells can be accelerated by the action of IL-4 or IL-10 and retarded by the action of IL-12 or IFN-F. The overwhelming fate of primed T cells is death by apoptosis, but a small number revert to the stable $CD45RA^F$ state, which prevents depopulation of the naïve T cell pool. Cells can be rescued from cytokine deprivation and actively-induced apoptosis by the action of either IL-2R F-chain cytdk ines, or by type-I interferons (see Fig 2).

these highly differentiated $CD45RB^{dull}$ cells selectively lose the capacity to synthesise IL-2, a cytokine which is particularly effective in preventing T cell apoptosis and also, to a lesser extent IFN-γ. This leads to the apoptosis of primed $CD45RB^{dull}$ cells, when they are stimulated in the absence of exogenous IL-2 [37]. This process is likely to be an important mechanism contributing to the maintenance of T cell homeostasis *in vivo*, preventing excessive increase in the size of the immune system.

Rheumatoid synovial T cells are very highly differentiated

T lymphocytes from the synovial fluid of patients with rheumatoid arthritis represent an extreme limit of differentiation. These cells express higher levels of CD45RO and lower levels of CD45RB than any cells found in the blood of the same patients [25]. RA blood T cells are very similar to healthy controls in this respect although here also there is a slightly increased proportion of highly differentiated cells in rheumatoid patients. It is currently unclear whether cells are recruited to the synovium in a recently primed $CD45RB^{bright}$ state, in a highly differentiated $CD45RB^{dull}$ state, or indeed whether any such selectivity occurs at all. However in recent experiments we have shown that $CD45RB^{dull}$ cells preferentially cross endothelial barriers *in vitro*, suggesting that $CD45RB^{dull}$ cells may be specifically recruited to inflammatory lesions [38]. The highly differentiated $CD45RB^{dull}$ character of rheumatoid synovial T cells explains many of the apparent functional discrepancies reported for this population, such as poor proliferative responses to stimulation and limited cytokine production [11], because peripheral blood $CD45RB^{dull}$ T cells behave in a very similar way [37].

As rheumatoid synovial T cells are very highly differentiated, we would expect them to be very susceptible to apoptosis and unstable, a process that should contribute towards resolution of inflammatory lesions. Yet T cells in the rheumatoid synovium show no evidence of apoptosis, using any currently available techniques [39] We eliminated the possibility that synovial T cells in RA are intrinsically resistant to apoptosis, because these cells die spontaneously and quite rapidly when cultured *in vitro* without any stimulus. Another possibility was that the cells did indeed apoptose, but were phagocytosed rapidly, before we could detect them. Macrophages recognise apoptotic T cells using the αVβ3 integrin-CD36 structure [40,41]. An alternative recognition structure expressed by all apoptotic cells is surface exposure of phosphatidyl-serine [42]. This molecule appears not to be used by macrophages during phagocytosis of apoptotic T cells [40], but detection of phosphatidyl-serine exposure using the serum protein Annexin V is a useful tool that allows us to identify apoptotic cells at least as early as phagocytes can [39,42]. We found no evidence of phosphatidyl-serine exposure on synovial T cells in RA. However, in most rheumatoid synovial samples, apoptotic neutrophils were readily detected, suggesting that the methods used were very sensitive [39]. An intriguing serendipitous observation confirmed that phagocytosis of apoptotic T cells was not a likely explanation for our failure to detect apoptosis of T cells in RA synovium: patients with acute uric acid crystal-induced arthritis actually show very high levels of T cell apoptosis *in vivo*. We found up to three-quarters of the T cells in these patients' synovia to be apoptotic [39]. This might explain the neutrophil dominance of these acute inflammatory lesions. So why should chronic rheumatoid inflammation be different? Could this apparent failure to remove lymphoid cells be involved in the process of chronic inflammation itself?

The regulation of T cell apoptosis by γ-chain cytokines and stromal cells.

Apoptosis of T cells can be induced actively by ligation of molecules such as Fas/Apo-1 (CD95) [43,44] or passively, by inadequate levels of stimulatory cytokines [45,46]. Previous reports have shown genes such as *Bcl-2* can prevent apoptosis, either through altering cell cycle rates or by anti-oxidant associated mechanisms [47-50]. Products of a related gene, *Bcl-x* can be differentially spliced to generate large ($Bcl\text{-}x_L$) and small ($Bcl\text{-}x_S$) mRNA transcripts which code for proteins that either prevent or induce apoptosis respectively [51]. In humans, no $Bcl\text{-}x_S$ protein has been detected; $Bcl\text{-}x_L$ is the only protein observed [52]. Bcl-2 and $Bcl\text{-}x_L$ appear to repress a common pathway leading to apoptosis [53]. We found that although Bcl-2 expression was low in synovial T cells, $Bcl\text{-}x_L$ remained at levels comparable to those seen in peripheral blood lymphocytes from the same patients [39]. This suggested that one reason for the lack of apoptosis in synovial T cells may be maintenance of high Bcl-x_L expression. This observation also indicated that factors present in the synovial microenvironment could differentially regulate Bcl-x_L expression relative to Bcl-2. In accord with this observation, T cells from gout patients who showed significant in situ apoptosis expressed low levels of both Bcl-2 and Bcl-x_L.

We have previously described two mechanisms by which apoptosis of cytokine deprived T cells can be retarded. When IL-2 is withdrawn from T cells the expression of both Bcl-2 and Bcl-x_L which are inhibitors of apoptosis falls sharply, while expression of apoptosis promoters such as Bax (an inhibitory ligand for Bcl-2) or Fas does not change significantly [52]. If T cells are subsequently cultured with any member of a class of cytokines that use the shared γ-chain signalling component of the IL-2 receptor (including IL-2, IL-4, IL-7, IL-13 and IL-15) apoptosis is prevented and Bcl-2 and Bcl-x_L expression are upregulated, indicating that these cytokines co-ordinate the expression of these genes [52]. The second mechanism for rescue involves co-culture of the T cells with fibroblast monolayers; this system induced survival without proliferation. An important observation was that Bcl-2 expression was reduced during fibroblast mediated rescue, but Bcl-x_L expression was maintained, indicating that this mechanism of survival uncouples the expression of these genes [46,54].

Although early reports suggested significant quantities of IL-15 to be present in rheumatoid synovium [55] more recent data from the same group suggests that the original values were an over-estimate by several orders of magnitude [56]. The limited T cell proliferation observed in situ and the low Bcl-2 expression observed suggest that IL-2R γ-chain cytokines are unlikely to be the principle mechanism preventing apoptosis of T cells in the rheumatoid joint [39]. However, the low Bcl-2 but high Bcl-x_L expression of the synovial T cells *in vivo* suggests that the stromal cell mediated route of rescue is likely to operate *in vivo*. Culture experiments *in vitro* supported this possibility and showed that co-culture with fibroblast-conditioned medium maintained the *in vivo* phenotype of synovial T cells (Bcl-2^{low}, Bcl-x_L^{high}). In contrast, addition of IL-15 led to high Bcl-2 and Bcl-x_L expression. Proliferating pannus tissue in rheumatoid joints contains a high density of fibroblasts [57], but synovial thickening in patients with acute crystal-induced-arthritis is usually much less marked or even absent, with considerably less evidence of fibroblast proliferation. Synovial T cells from patients with gout could be rescued by either IL-15 or fibroblast conditioned medium, but the phenotype produced was in each case that predicted, i.e. IL-15 induced Bcl-2^{high}Bcl-x_L^{high} and stromal rescue induced a Bcl-2^{low}Bclx_L^{high} phenotype. However, gout T cells *in vivo* express a Bcl-2^{low}Bcl-x_L^{low} phenotype and die by apoptosis. These results suggest strongly that apoptosis of T cells in the rheumatoid synovium is actively inhibited by stromal cells present in the proliferating pannus tissue.

Stromal mediators of survival

So what is it that the inflammatory microenvironment stromal cells provide to keep T cells alive? Hyaluronic acid is present in extremely high levels in synovial fluid; intriguingly this molecule has been reported to block Fas-mediated activation-induced apoptosis in mouse T cell hybridomas [58]. Unfortunately for those of us who like elegant solutions, hyaluronic acid does not inhibit spontaneous synovial T cell apoptosis *in vitro* [39]. This does not necessarily exclude an active role for hyaluronate in modulating activation-induced apoptosis in situ, as the Fas derived signals generated are likely to be transient and not persist in culture [53]. Many integin molecules bind to specific ligands through a motif consisting of Arg-Gly-Asp [60]. *In vitro* the peptide Arg-Gly-Asp-Ser (RGDS) has been used to inhibit such interactions for many years; Arg-Gly-Glu-Ser (RGES) is used as a control. We showed that the ability of fibroblast conditioned medium to rescue synovial T cells from apoptosis was markedly "inhibited" by the RGDS but not the RGES peptide, suggesting that an integrin interaction was likely to be involved [39]. This is actually completely wrong. We have now shown that the effect of RGD peptides in biological experiments is almost exclusively independent of integrins. The peptides enter cells directly, bind to caspase 3 and induce a conformational change that leads to the autocatalytic cleavage of this molecule [63]. Caspase 3 plays a pivotal role in the effector stage of apoptosis, analogous in many respects to C3 in the complement cascade. Not surprisingly RGD peptides directly induce apoptosis in target cells. While this observation considerably alters our perception of adhesion molecule biology, it also suggests a very powerful therapeutic tool. RGD peptides have been used in preliminary therapeutic trials, intended to target adhesion and migration of cells in tumour metastasis, angiogenesis and several related conditions. Intriguingly, the effects of these peptides were dramatic, even at doses too low to significantly affect integrin function, and the effects persisted after the peptides had been cleared. It seems very likely that what was detected in these experiments was induction of apoptosis.

So what is it in stromal cells that keeps T cells alive? Interferon-β [64]. We have now shown that both α and β interferons are capable of maintaining T cell survival. Inhibitory antibody and cell signalling experiments suggest that only interferon-β is produced by fibroblasts in sufficient quantity to affect survival. Interferon-α is a prominent product of macrophages, which of course make up about half of pannus tissue. We have shown that these cytokines are abundant in rheumatoid, but not in acute inflammatory synovium, and also that the cells at these sites appear to have been rescued by their actions. The identification of type-I interferons as the principle agent for survival enabled us to study its effects on other cells in the synovial microenvironment. We found that its effects are not restricted to T cells. Neutrophil survival and also fibroblast survival is extended markedly by its action. The stromal-mediated rescue of T cells appears to be a fundamental process in the generation and maintenance of T cell memory, providing the only currently known mechanism for inducing a resting G0/G1 state in activated T cells, without apoptosis. Precisely the same mechanism under certain circumstances induces persistence of chronic inflammatory cells.

The mechanism by which type-I interferons prolong survival seems to be complex. Many cytokine receptors are closely related and are associated with one or more members of the JAK family of tyrosine kinases [65]. JAKs couple cytokine receptors to a variety of signalling proteins including Ras, PI-3-kinase, PLC-γ and the Stat family of transcription factors. Jak-1 kinase interacts specifically with the IL-2R β-chain while Jak-3 interacts with the γ-chain, activating the STAT-5 transcription factor [66]. We have shown that the signalling pathway employed by IFN-β in upregulating Bcl-x_L in T cells is through dimerisation of STAT-1 and activation of the IRES-STAT complex. The latter is completely specific for type-I interferons. We identified a putative STAT binding sequence in the Bcl-x gene regulatory sequence, and have now shown that this interacts with the IFN-induced IRES complex, leading to transcription activation [Pilling, Girdlestone & Salmon – Manuscript in Preparation]. The specific induction of STAT-1 and IRES complexes by fibroblast conditioned medium was mimicked by synovial fluid [64] suggesting that this is a key mechanism in the rescue of synovial cells from apoptosis. Intriguingly, no STAT-5 inducing signals were identified, which would have been the expected mechanism for γ-chain cytokines such as IL-15.

There is however a problem with the STAT-1/Bcl-x pathway as the principal mediator of rescue from apoptosis. It is too slow. Activation of STATs and translocation to the nucleus takes about 15 minutes [64]. Transcription, processing and translation of the gene product will then take several hours before functional Bcl-x_L protein can successfully inhibit apoptosis. Yet IFN-β prevents Fas-mediated apoptosis when added at the initiation of the induction process [64]. Fas-mediated apoptosis proceeds too quickly to be blocked by the Bcl-x_L induction route. Furthermore IFN-β also retards neutrophil apoptosis, with a significant delay to apoptosis seen within 3 hours and prior to any detectable changes in Bcl-x expression. The STAT-1/IRES pathway therefore appears to be fundamentally a key mechanism for reducing susceptibility to apoptosis, not for blocking its effector function.

Our current understanding of intra-cellular signalling events involved in the regulation of apoptosis suggests that there are several distinct or "private" pathways that converge to effect a common apoptotic programme [67]. A majority of these pathways can be regulated downstream by members of the bcl-2 family of proteins. An alternative and much more rapid route for inhibition of apoptosis by IFN-β may lie in the direct modulation of one or more of these pathways. We are currently investigating the involvement of a PI3 kinase dependent pathway in the interferon-mediated rescue of T-cells and neutrophils from apoptosis. AKT is a serine/ threonine kinase that plays a central role in the regulation of apoptosis [68]. It is activated through a PI3 kinase dependent pathway [69]. AKT deactivates the pro-apoptotic member of the bcl-2 family BAD by phosphorylation [70]. AKT also phosphorylates a range of other molecules, including transcription factors of the forkhead family [71], which are involved in the regulation of transcription of proapoptotic genes, such as FAS-L. Recently, AKT was also implicated in the regulation of caspase activation, by phosphorylating of caspase 9, preventing its activation [72]. Caspase 9 is involved in the induction of apoptosis through the mitochondrial pathway [73]. Many apoptotic signals, such as FAS receptor crosslinking, irradiation and staurosporine lead to release of cytochrome c from the mitochondria. In the cytosol, cytochrome c binds to APAF1 and procaspase 9. Formation of this complex, known as the apoptosome, leads to proteolytic activation of caspase 9, which then cleaves and activates caspase 3. Caspase 3 cleaves a large number of target proteins within the cell and thus leads to many of the characteristic features of apoptosis, like DNA cleavage and nuclear condensation. Phosphorylation of caspase 9 on serine[196] by the serine threonine kinase Akt prevents the proteolytic activation of caspase 9 and its subsequent activation of Caspase 3 [73]. We are currently investigating the effects of IFN-β on AKT activation and subsequent events. This pathway appears to provide a rapid upstream mechanism for the active inhibition of apoptosis by interferon.

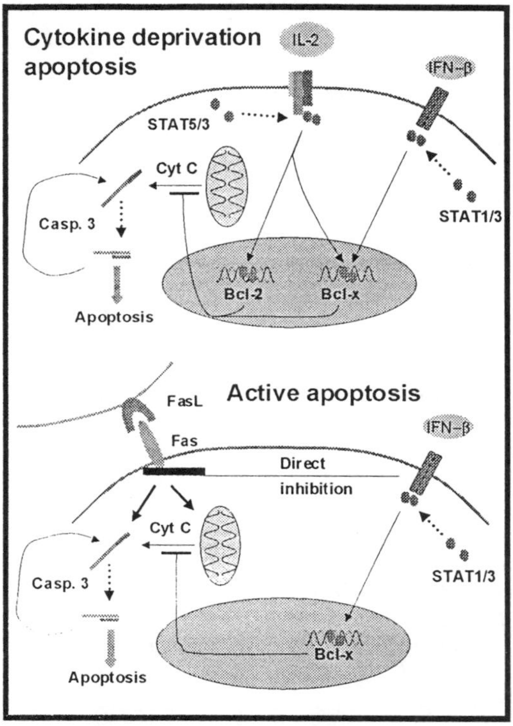

Figure 2. Mechanisms of T cell rescue from apoptosis. Both IL-2R γ-chain cytokines and type-I IFNs can inhibit cytokine deprivation-induced apoptosis by induction of BCL-2 family members (Bcl-2/Bcl-x_L). These molecules act by preventing the release of cytochrome-c from the mitochondria. This inhibits formation of the apoptosome and therefore, cleavage of caspase 3. This process is too slow to block Fas induced apoptosis, so alternative, upstream mechanisms must also operate.

Protein kinase C (PKC) regulates a large number of intracellular signalling events, including cell proliferation and apoptosis, with its pleiotropic actions mediated by the distinct actions of the 11 isoenzymes of PKC [74]. Three such isoforms PKCα, PKCβll and PKCδ appear to actively regulate apoptosis. The first two inhibit apoptosis, while active PKCδ induces apoptosis [75]. We deprived T-cells of survival factors and after varying intervals fractionated the cells into their cytoplasmic, membrane and cytoskeletal constituents. Translocation of PKC to membrane or cytoskeletal compartments is an indicator of enzyme activation. Western blot analysis showed that PKC delta accumulated in the cytoskeletal fraction in the early stages of apoptosis [76]. Addition of IFN-β inhibited this translocation. Immunofluorescence staining of cytospin preparations indicated that in the early stages of apoptosis PKC delta accumulated at the nuclear envelope. This is consistent with previous data suggesting that the primary target for PKC-δ is Lamin B [77], a cytoskeletal component of the nuclear envelope. Addition of IFN-β to T-cells already deprived of survival factors showed a rapid retranslocation of PKC-δ to the cytoplasm, suggesting that this is a reversible step in the signalling pathway to apoptosis. PKC-δ can also be activated by proteolytic degradation by caspase 3, which releases the catalytic (40kDa) fragment from the control of the regulatory domain. IFN-β also actively inhibited the downstream activation of PKC-δ by caspase 3. Interestingly, preliminary data also revealed that IFN-β induced translocation of PKC-α and this may contribute to T cell survival [77]. Furthermore, inhibition of neutrophil apoptosis by IFN-β was also associated with a delay in the appearance of caspase activated PKC-δ. These results suggest at least a bi-modal signalling route for the regulation of apoptosis by type-I interferons and also that PKC isoenzymes offer a potential therapeutic target in the control of rheumatoid arthritis and other forms of chronic inflammation.

Infiltrating T cells persist in chronic inflammation through active suppression of apoptosis by stromal cells.

The available data suggest that T cells in the rheumatoid synovium are a perfectly normal population of very highly differentiated cells. Our results suggest that the inflammatory T cell infiltrate persists principally because apoptosis is actively suppressed by the synovial microenvironment [39]. It is very unlikely that T cell apoptosis is completely blocked. We suggest that during active flares of rheumatoid disease activity, probably associated with random infections, cells are actively recruited to the joint in a largely non-specific manner. During more stable periods of disease, the suppression of T cell apoptosis will maintain the infiltrating population for extended periods of time. The stromal (IFN-β) mediated rescue of activated T cells from apoptosis is essentially a physiological mechanism for the generation and maintenance of T cell memory, that under certain circumstances is subverted to the perpetuation of chronic inflammation. These mechanism prevent the death of infiltrating inflammatory cells of many types, not just T cells. Intriguingly, spontaneous neutrophil apoptosis is also strongly retarded (Wang, Scheel-Toellner, Salmon and Lord – in preparation). The next clear question has to be: "why don't the cells simply migrate out from the lesion when the input stimulus is lost?" The answer to this appears to be active upregulation of specific chemokine receptors by the synovial microenvironment (Buckley, Amft, Lord Akbar and Salmon, submitted).

It is unclear at the moment whether synovial pannus formation is a semi-neoplastic process of self-driven proliferation of fibroblasts, or is itself a product of the chronic inflammatory process [61]. However, it seems wise to be cautious in proposing a fundamental defect in synovial fibroblasts as the likely cause of the rheumatoid lesion at this stage. Chronic inflammation in many respects is a very similar process wherever it is found. In our studies we have compared rheumatoid arthritis patients with uric acid-induced crystal arthritis, but chronic and acute inflammation may be more appropriate labels, because the characteristic of persistence sustained by interaction of immune cells with the stromal microenvironment is likely to be a feature of all chronic inflammation. Inflammatory T cell infiltrates are not cleared by apoptosis in patients with a range of chronic inflammatory myopathies. We would suggest that these cells like those in the rheumatoid synovium may actually receive positive signals to stay alive. The role of the inflammatory fibroblast in perpetuating the immunological aspects of chronic inflammation deserves considerable attention, and offers important new approaches for treating these intractable diseases.

References

1. Kearney, E.R., Walunas, T.L., Karr, R.W., Morton, P.A., Loh, D.Y., Bluestone, J.A. & Jenkins, M.K. "Antigen-dependent clonal expansion of a trace population of antigen specific CD4+ T cells *in vivo* is dependent on CD28 costimulation and inhibited by CTLA-4." *J. Immunol.* 1995; **155**: 1032-1036.
2. Ahmed, R. & Gray, D. "Immunological memory and protective immunity - understanding their relation." *Science* 1996; **272**: 54-60.
3. Tough, D.F., Borrow, P. & Sprent, J. Induction of bystander T cell proliferation by viruses and type I interferon *in vivo*. *Science* 1996; **272**: 1947-1950.
4. Callan, M.F.C., Steven, J., Krausa, P., Wilson, J.D.K., Moss, P.A.H., Gillespie, G.M., Bell, J.I., Rickinson, A.B. & McMichael, A.J. "Large clonal expansions of CD8+ T cells in acute infectious mononucleosis." *Nature Medicine* 1996; **2**: 906-911.
5. Nagata, S. & Golstein, P. "The Fas death factor." *Science* 1995; **267**: 1449-1456.
6. Tough, D.F. & Sprent, J. "Viruses and T cell turnover - evidence for bystander proliferation." *Immunol. Rev.*. 1996; **150**: 129-142.
7. Akbar, A.N. & Salmon, M. "Cellular environments and apoptosis: tissue microenvironments control activated T cell death." *Immunol. Today* 1997; **18**: 72-76.
8. Akbar, A.N., Borthwick, N., Salmon, M., Gombert, W., Bofill, M., Shamsadeen, N., Pilling, D., Pett, S., Grundy, J.E. & Janossy, G. "The significance of low Bcl-2 expression by CD45RO T cells in normal individuals and patients with acute viral infections. The role of apoptosis in T cell memory." *J. Exp. Med.* 1993; **178**: 427-438.
9. Orteu, C.H., Poulter, L.W., Rustin, M.H.A., Sabin, C.A., Salmon, M. & Akbar, A.N. "The role of apoptosis in the resolution of T cell mediated cutaneous inflammation." *J.Immunol.* 1998; **161**: 1619-1629.
10. Salmon M (1992) "The immunogenetic componant of susceptibility to rheumatoid arthritis.*Current Opinion in Rheumatology 4, 342-347*
11. Salmon M; Gaston JSH "The role of T lymphocytes in rheumatoid arthritis" Br Med Bull. 1995; **51**, *332-345*
12. Kitas GD, Salmon M, Farr M, Young SP, Bacon PA. "T cell functional defects in RA: intrinsic or extrinsic." J. Autoimmunity. 1988; **1**: 339-51.
13. Panayi GS, Lanchbury JS, Kingsley GH. "The importance of the T-cell in initiating and maintaining the chronic synovitis of rheumatoid-arthritis" Arthritis Rheum. 1992; **35**: 729-735.
14. Firestein GS, Zvaifler NJ. "How important are T cells in chronic rheumatoid synovitis?" Arthritis Rheum 1990; **33** :768-773.
15. Wordsworth BP, Lanchbury JSS, Sakkas LI, Welsh KI, Panayi GS, Bell JI. "HLA-DR4 subtype frequencies in rheumatoid-arthritis indicate that DRB1 is the major susceptibility locus within the HLA class-II region." Proc Natn Acad Sci USA 1989 **86** 10049-53
16. WinchesterRJ, Gregerson PK. "The molecular-basis of susceptibility to rheumatoid-arthritis – the conformational equivalence hypothesis." Springer Semin Immunopathol 1988 **10**, 119-139
17. Salmon M. "The immunogenetic componant of susceptibility to rheumatoid arthritis." *Current Opinion in Rheumatology* 1992 **4**, 342-347
18. De Jongh BM, Van Romunde LKJ, Valkenburg HA, De Lange GG, Van Rood JJ. Epidemiological-study of HLA and GM in rheumatoid-arthritis and related symptoms in an open dutch population." Ann Rheum Dis 1984 **43**, 613-619
19. Salmon M; Emery P; Wordsworth BP; Tunn EJ; Bacon PA, Bell JI. "HLA Dw4 is associated with persistence rather than the induction of rheumatoid arthritis." *Br J. Rheumatol* 1993 *32 628-630*

20. Gough A, Faint J, Salmon M, Hassell A, Wordsworth P, Pilling D, Birley A, Emery P. "Genetic typing of patients with inflammatory arthritis at presentation is predictive of outcome." *Arthritis Rheum* 1994 **34**, 1166-1170

21. Van Zeben D, Hazes LMW, Zwinderman AH, Cats A, Schreuder GMT, D'Amaro J, Breedveld FC. "Association of HLA-DR4 with a more progressive disease course in patients with rheumatoid-arthritis - results of a follow-up-study." Arthritis Rheum 1991 **34**, 822-830

22. Wordsworth P, Pile K, Buckley JD, Lanchbury JSS, Ollier B, Lathrop M, Bell JI. "HLA heterozygosity contributes to susceptibility to rheumatoid-arthritis." Am J. Hum Genet 1992 **51**, 585-591

23. Arnett F.C., S.M. Edworthy, D.A. Bloch, D.J. Mcshane, J.F. Fries, N.S. Cooper, L.A. Healey, S.R. Kaplan, M.H. Liang, H.S. Luthra, T.A. Medsger, D.M. Mitchell, D.H. Neustadt, R.S. Pinals, J.G. Schaller, J.T. Sharp, R.L. Wilder, G.G.Hunder. "The American-Rheumatism-Association 1987 revised criteria for the classification of rheumatoid-arthritis." *Arthritis Rheum.* 1988. **31**:315-324.

24. Uematsu, Y., Wege, H., Straus, A., Ott, M., Bannwarth, W., Lanchbury, J., Panayi, G., and Steinmetz, M. "The T-cell-receptor repertoire in the synovial-fluid of a patient with rheumatoid-arthritis is polyclonal." *Proc Natn Acad Sci USA* 1991; **88**: 8534-8538.

25. Pluschke, G., Ricken, G., Taube, H., Kroninger, S., Melchers, I., Peter, H.H., Eichmann, K., and Krawinkel, U. "Biased T-cell receptor v-alpha region repertoire in the synovial-fluid of rheumatoid-arthritis patients." *Eur J. Immunol* 1991; **21**: 2749-2754.

26. Fischer, H.P., Sharrock, C.E.M., Colston, M.J., and Panayi, G.S. "Limiting dilution analysis of proliferative T-cell responses to mycobacterial 65-KDa heat-shock protein fails to show significant frequency differences between synovial-fluid and peripheral-blood of patients with rheumatoid-arthritis." *Eur J. Immunol* 1991 **21**: 2937-2941.

27. Marguerie, C., Lunardi, C., and So, A "PCR-based analysis of the Tcr repertoire in human autoimmune- diseases." *Immunology Today* 1992; **13**:336-338.

28. Pelton BK, Harvey AR Denman_AM "The rheumatoid synovial-membrane participates in systemic anti- viral immune-responses." Clin Exp Immunol 1985 **62**, 657-661

29. Sun, J.B., Link, H., Olsson, T., Xiao, B.G., Andersson, G., Ekre, H.P., Linington, C., and Diener, P. "T-cell and B-cell responses to myelin-oligodendrocyte glycoprotein in multiple-sclerosis." *J. Immunol* 1991; **146**:1490-1495.

30. Offner, H., Buenafe, A.C., Vainiene, M., Celnik, B., Weinberg, A.D., Gold, D.P., Hashim, G., and Vandenbark, A.A. "Where, when, and how to detect biased expression of disease- relevant V-beta-genes in rats with experimental autoimmune encephalomyelitis." *J. Immunol* 1993; **151**:506-517.

31. Paulus HE; Machleder HI; Levine S; Yu DTY; McDonald NS "Lymphocyte involvement in rheumatoid arthritis." Arthritis Rheum. 1977; **20**.1249-1262

32. Karsh J; Klippel JH; Plotz PH; Decker JL; Wright DG; Flye MV "Lymphophoresis in rheumatoid arthritis." Arthritis Rheum 1981; **24**, 867-873

33. Aaron S; Paetku V: Clin. Exp. "synovial cell secretion of Il-2 in vitro, a limiting dilution analysis." Rheumatol 1991; **9**, 113-118

34. Pitzalis C, Kingsley GH, Covelli M, Meliconi R, Markey A, Panayi Gs "Selective migration of the human helper-inducer memory T-cell subset - confirmation by in vivo cellular kinetic-studies." *Eur. J. Immunol* 1991; **21**: 369-76.

35. Matthews, N., Emery, P., Pilling, D., Akbar, A., and Salmon, M "CD45RB exon expression by T lymphocytes from patients with rheumatoid arthritis." Arthritis Rheum. 1993; **36**: 603-607

36. Mackay, C.R., Marston, W.L., and Dudler, L. "Naive and memory T-cells show distinct pathways of lymphocyte recirculation." *J.Exp.Med.* 1990; **171**:801-817.

37. Salmon, M., D. Pilling, N.J. Borthwick, N. Viner, G. Janossy, P.A. Bacon, and A.N. Akbar. "The progressive differentiation of primed T cells is associated with an increasing susceptibility to apoptosis." *Eur. J. Immunol* 1994; **24**: 892-899.

38. Borthwick NJ, Akbar AN, MacCormac LP, Lowdell M, Craigen JL, Hassan I, Grundy JE, Salmon M, Yong KL "Selective migration of highly differentiated primed T cells, defined by low expression of CD45RB, across human umbilical vein endothelial cells: Effects of viral infection on transmigration ." *Immunology* 1997 **90,** 272-280

39. Salmon M, Scheel-Toellner D, Huissoon AP, Pilling D, Shamsadeen N, Hyde H, Dangeac AD, Bacon PA, Emery P and Akbar AN "Inhibition of T cell apoptosis in the rheumatoid synovium." *J. Clin Invest.* 1997; **99**: 439-446

40. Akbar, A.N., J. Savill, W. Gombert, M. Bofill, N.J. Borthwick, F. Whitelaw, J. Grundy, G. Janossy, and M. Salmon. "The specific recognition by macrophages of $CD8^+CD45RO^+$ T cells undergoing apoptosis: a mechanism for T cell clearance during resolution of viral infections." *J.Exp.Med.* 1994 **180**: 1943-1947.

41. Savill, J., V. Fadok, P. Henson, and C. Haslett. "Phagocyte recognition of cells undergoing apoptosis." *Immunol Today* 1993; **14**:131-136.

42. Martin S.J, C.P.M. Reutelingsperger, A.J. Mcgahon, J.A. Rader, R.C.A.A. Vanschie, D.M. Laface, D.R. Green. "Early redistribution of plasma-membrane phosphatidylserine is a general feature of apoptosis regardless of the initiating stimulus - inhibition by overexpression of bcl-2 and abl." *J.Exp.Med.* 1995; **182:** 1545-1556.

43. Dhein, J., H. Walczak, C. Baumler, K.M. Debatin, and P.H. Krammer. "Autocrine T cell suicide mediated by Apo-1/(Fas/CD95)." *Nature* 1995; **373**: 438-441.

44. Brunner, T., R.J. Mogil, D. Laface, N.J. Yoo, A. Mahboubi, F. Echeverri, S.J. Martin, W.R. Force, D.H. Lynch, C.F. Ware, and D.R. Green. "Cell-autonomous fas (CD95) Fas-ligand interaction mediates activation-induced apoptosis in t-cell hybridomas." *Nature* 1995; **373**: 441-444.

45. Cohen J.J, R.C. Duke, V.A. Fadok, and K.S. Sellins. "Apoptosis and programmed cell-death in immunity." *Ann. Rev. Immunol* 1992; **10**: 267-293.

46. Akbar, A.N., N. Borthwick, M. Salmon, W. Gombert, M. Bofill, N. Shamsadeen, D. Pilling, S. Pett, J.E. Grundy, and G. Janossy. "The significance of low bcl-2 expression by CD45RO-T-cells in normal individuals and patients with acute viral-infections - The role of apoptosis in T-cell memory." *J.Exp.Med.* 1993; **178:** 427-438.

47. Mazel S; Burtrum D; Petrie HT J. "Regulation of cell division cycle progression by bcl-2 expression: A potential mechanism for inhibition of programmed cell death." Exp Med. 1996; **183**, 2219-2226

48. O'Reilly LA; Huang DCS; Strasser A "The cell death inhibitor Bcl-2 and its homologues influence control of cell cycle entry." EMBO J. 1996; **15**, 6979-6990

49. Korsmeyer, S.J., Shutter, J.R., Veis, D.J., Merry, D.E., and Oltvai, Z.N "Bcl-2/bax - a rheostat that regulates an antioxidant pathway and cell-death." *Seminars In Cancer Biology* 1993; **4**: 327-332,

50. Hyde H, Salmon M, Janossy G & Akbar AN Upregulation of intracellular glutathione by fibroblast-derived factors: prevention of activated T cell apoptosis in the presence of low Bcl-2. *Blood* 1997; **89**: 2453-2460

51. Boise, L.H., M. Gonzalezgarcia, C.E. Postema, L.Y. Ding, T. Lindsten, L.A. Turka, X.H. Mao, G. Nunez, and C.B. Thompson. "Bcl-x, a bcl-2-related gene that functions as a dominant regulator of apoptotic cell-death." *Cell* 1993; **74**: 597-608.

52. Akbar A.N., N. Borthwick, R.G. Wickremasinghe, P. Panayiotidis, P D. illing, M.. Bofill, S. Krajewski, J.C. Reed, M. Salmon. "Interleukin-2 receptor common γ-chain cytokines regulate activated T cell apoptosis in response to growth factor withdrawal: selective induction of anti-apoptotic (bcl-2, bcl-x_L) but not pro-apoptotic (bax, bcl-x_S) gene expression." *Eur J. Immunol,* 1996; **26**: 294-299

53. Hale A.J, C.A. Smith, L.C. Sutherland, V.E.A. Stoneman, V.L. Longthorne, A.C. Culhane, G.T. Williams. "Apoptosis - Molecular regulation of cell death." *Eur. J Biochem.* 1996; **236**: 1-26.

54. Gombert, W., D.L. Wallace, N.J. Borthwick, H. Hyde, D. Pilling, M. Bofill, P.C.L. Beverley, G. Janossy, M. Salmon, and A.N. Akbar. "Fibroblasts prevent apoptosis of IL-2 deprived T cells without inducing proliferation: a selective effect on Bcl-x_L expression." *Immunology* 1996; **86**, 397-404

55. McInnes, I.B., J. Al-Mughales, M. Field, B.P. Leung, F.P. Huang, R. Dixon, R.D. Sturrock, P.C. Wilkinson, and F.Y. Liew "The role of interleukin-15 in T cell migration and activation in rheumatoid arthritis." *Nature Med.,* 1996; **2**: 175-182.

56. McInnes IB, Leung BP, Sturrock RD, Field M, Liew FY "Interleukin 15 mediates T cell dependent regulation of tumor necrosis factor alpha production in rheumatoid arthritis." Nature Med. 1997 **3**, 189-95

57. Fassbender HG. "Pathology of rheumatic diseases." New York: Springer-Verlag Inc., 1975

58. Ayroldi E, L. Cannarile, G. Migliorati, A. Bartoli, I. Nicoletti, C. Riccardi "CD44 (Pgp-1) inhibits CD3 and dexamethasone-induced apoptosis." Blood: 1995; **86:** 2672-2678.

59. Yokota K, Murata N, Saiko O, Shimizu M, Springer TA, Kishimoto T. "High avidity state of leukocyte function-associated antigen-1 on rheumatoid synovial-fluid T-lymphocytes." J. Immunol. 1995; **155,** 4118-24

60. Stewart M., M. Thiel, and N. Hogg. "Leukocyte integrins." *Curr. Opin. Cell Biol.* 1995; **7:** .690-696.

61. Firestein GS "Invasive fibroblast-like synoviocytes in rheumatoid-arthritis -passive responders or transformed aggressors." Arthritis Rheum 1996; **39**, 1781-1790

62. Schneider C; Gold R; Dalakas MC, Schmied M; Lassmann H; Toyks KV; Hartung H-P "MHC Class-I mediated cytotoxicity does not induce apoptosis in muscle fibres nor in inflammatory T cells - Studies in patients with polymyositis, dermatomyositis and inclusion body myositis." J. Neurophathol Exp Neurol. 1996; **55,** 1205-1209

63. Buckley CD, Pilling D, Henriquez NV, Parsonage G, Threlfall K, Scheel-Toellner D, Simmons DL, Akbar AN, Lord JM, Salmon M – "RGD peptides induce apoptosis by direct caspase-3 activation: a ubiquitous motif for cell death" *Nature* 1999; **397**: 534-53964.

64. Pilling D, Akbar AN, Girdlestone J, Orteu CH, Borthwick NJ, Amft N Scheel-Toellner D, Buckley CD, Salmon M "Interferon-β is the principle mediator of stromal cell rescue of T cells from apoptosis." *Eur J. Immunol* 1999; **29**: 1041-1050.

66. Salmon M; Pilling D; Mappin C and Akbar AN "Human T cell differentiation and cytokine regulation." in *Haemopoeitic Cell Growth Factors* ed. Gordon & Whetton. Plenum *Blood Cell Biochemistry* 1996; **7**, 203-215

67. Taher TEI, Smit L, Griffioen AW, SchilderTol EJM, Borst J, Pals ST "Signaling through CD44 is mediated by tyrosine kinases - Association with p56(lck) in T lymphocytes." *J.Biol.Chem.* 1996; **171:** 2863.

68. Hale AJ, Smith CA, Sutherland LC, Stoneman VEA, Longthorne VL, Culhane AC, Williams GT "Apoptosis - Molecular regulation of cell death." *Eur. J. Biochem* 1996; **236**: 1

69. Downward_J "Mechanisms and consequences of activation of protein kinase B/Akt." *Curr. Opin. Cell Biol*, 1998 ;**10**: 262-267

70. Toker, A., and Cantley, L. "Signalling through the lipid products of phosphoinositide-3-OH kinase." *Nature*. 1997; **387**: 673-676

71. Datta, S.R., Dudek, H., Tao X., Masters, S, Fu, H., Gotoh, Y., and Greenberg, M. "AKT phosphorylation of BAD couples survival signals to the cell-intrinsic death machinery." *Cell* 1997; **91**:231-241.

72. Brunet, A., Bonni, A., Zigmond, M. J., Lin, M.Z., Juo, P., Hu, L.S., Anderson, M.J. arden, K.C., Blenis, J. andGreenberg, M.E. "Akt promotes cell survival by phosphorylating and inhibiting a Forkhead transcription factor." *Cell*. 1999; **92**:857-868.

73. Cardone, M., Roy, N., Stennicke, H.R., Salvesen G.S., Franke, T. F., Stanbridge, E., Frisch, S. and Reed, J.C. "Regulation of cell death protease Caspase-9 by phosphorylation." *Science*, 1998; **282**:1318-1320.

74. Green, D.R and Reed, J.C. "Mitochondria and Apoptosis" *Science* 1998; **281**: 1309-1312.

75. Dekker LV, Parker PJ. "Protein-kinase-C - a question of specificity." *Trends Biochem Sci* 1994; **19**:73

76. Ghayur T, Hugunin M, Talanin RV, Ratnofsky S, Quinlan C, Emoto Y, Datta R, Kufe D. "Proteolytic activation of protein kinase C delta by an ICE/CED 3-like protease induces characteristics of apoptosis." *J.Exp.Med.* 1996; **184**: 2399

77. Scheel-Toellner D, Pilling D, Hardie D, Akbar AN, Salmon M, Lord JM "Inhibition of T-cell Apoptosis by Interferon-ß Reverses Nuclear Translocation of Protein kinase C-delta." *Eur J. Immunol – In Press.*

78. Lord JM, Garrone B, Griffiths G, Watters D. "Protein-kinase-C - a family of isoenzymes with distinct roles in pathogenesis." *J.Cell.Biochem.* 1995; **S19B**: 275.

79. Firestein G.S., M. Yeo, and N.J. Zvaifler. "Apoptosis in rheumatoid-arthritis synovium." *J. Clin. Invest.* 1995; **96**: 1631-1638.

80. Migita K, Eguchi K, Ichinose Y, Kawabe Y, Tsukada T, Aoyagi T, Nagataki S "Effects of rapamycin on apoptosis of rheumatoid synovial cells." *Clin Exp Immunol* 1997; **108**: 199-203

81. Okamoto K, Asahara H, Kobayashi T, Matsuno H, Hasunuma T, Kobata T, Sumida T, Nishioka K "Induction of apoptosis in the rheumatoid synovium by Fas ligand gene transfer." *Gene Therapy* 1998; **5:** 331-8

82. Firestein GS, Echeverri F, Yeo M, Zvaifler NJ, Green DR "Somatic mutations in the p53 tumor suppressor gene in rheumatoid arthritis synovium." *Proc Natn Acad Sci USA* 1997; **94:** 10895-10900

EUCAMBIS: Immunology and Ageing in Europe
G. Pawelec (Ed.)
IOS Press, 2000

Influence of Ageing on Human NK Cells

Erminia MARIANI and Andrea FACCHINI
Laboratorio di Immunologia e Genetica, Istituto di Ricerca Codivilla-Putti, IOR
Dipartimento di Medicina Interna e Gastroenterologia, Bologna University, Italy

Abstract. The pattern of the various age-related diseases suggests that the immune system is one of the most important targets of ageing. We demonstrated that despite the progressive increase in the number of peripheral NK cells found in the elderly, there was no corresponding increase in lytic activity. On the contrary, a decreased function of circulating NK cells from old subjects was observed after a sorting procedure or after limiting dilution and cloning of NK cell precursors. This decrease in function was not related to a reduced ability of old cells to form conjugates with targets nor to a modified amount or production of perforins in NK cell cytoplasm, but a significant impairment of lytic efficiency was shown on a per NK cell basis. In addition, we found a pronounced age-related decrease in the ability to generate total inositol phosphates and particularly inositol triphosphate by NK cells following K562 stimulation (spontaneous cytolytic activity), together with an attenuated and delayed hydrolysis of phosphoinositide biphosphate, while phosphoinositide turnover is preserved following Fc triggering (ADCC). Increasing evidence has demonstrated that the immune, endocrine and nervous systems are closely integrated and communicate through circulating cytokines, hormones and neurotransmitters. Many hormones have an important influence on the homeostasis of the immune system and in maintaining the integrity of body composition. NK cell number and cytolytic activity were significantly associated with serum concentrations of vitamin D. Anthropometric parameters indicating fat reserves and muscle reserves were also directly correlated with NK cell number and activity and fat indicators were linked to vitamin D. Because of the close interrelations between malnutrition and immunodeficiency, these results stress the paramount importance of nutritional evaluation in the clinical assessment of elderly people.

1. Definition of NK Cells

Natural Killer (NK) together with polymorphonuclear cells and macrophages are components of the natural immune system. NK cells, in particular, have a role in the development and regulation of immunosurveillance. They represent a primary host defence system because they are responsible for spontaneous killing of certain types of tumour cells and of virally infected cells [1]. NK activity has been found to be decreased in several diseases such as cancer [2], immunodeficiency disorders [3] autoimmune diseases [4], chronic fatigue syndrome [5] and is influenced by environmental conditions, mental stress [6] and physical exercise [7], lifestyle factors like smoking [8] and alcohol consumption [9] and, finally, by age [10].

NK cells have been described as "large granular lymphocytes" lacking T cell receptorsand characterised by the membrane expression of CD56 (N-CAM) and CD16 (Fcγ

RIII, low affinity receptor for IgG Fc fragment). These cells may also coexpress T cell markers like CD2, CD8, CD57, and some molecules involved in intercellular adhesion (CD11a, CD11b, CD18, CD54 and CD58). In addition, they display two alternative mechanisms of cytolysis: a direct spontaneous cytotoxicity against a variety of tumour cells and indirect Fc receptor-mediated cytotoxicity against antibody-coated targets (ADCC; Antibody-Dependent Cell-mediated Cytotoxicity) [1].

2. Selection of Elderly Subjects

The pattern of the various age-related diseases suggests that the immune system is one of the most important targets of ageing. Since advancing age in humans is associated with increased morbidity and mortality from neoplastic and infectious diseases [11], several groups have investigated the impact of ageing on the immune system [12] and on the mechanisms and surface structures involved in NK cell activation and function.

Immune responses in older people are less homogeneous than those in younger individuals; in particular nutritional deficiencies may have a major effect on immunocompetence and the ageing process [13, 14].

The selection criteria for the study population have been a major problem in immuno-gerontological studies leading to different results, probably due to the coexistence of pathological processes together with age-related physiological changes. The introduction of selection criteria for healthy subjects following the "Senieur " protocol was an important step in studying the immune system during ageing in order to avoid defects derived from underlying diseases or pharmacological interference and to study the ageing process under basal conditions [15]. This protocol, generally adopted by several groups studying immunogerontology, admits subjects who present normal biochemical and medical parameters and are not taking drugs or supplements known to influence the immune system (about 10-15% of aged subjects), therefore decreasing inter-individual variability of immunological parameters.

3. Distribution of NK Cells

In 1990 we demonstrated that the absolute and relative number of circulating NK cells progressively increases in the peripheral blood of healthy elderly people selected following the "Senieur" protocol [16] (Figure 1). In the age decades from 71 to 95 years, the number of NK cells was nearly doubled compared with a young population of 25-35 year old subjects (Figure 1), a finding confirmed by other groups [17, 18].

This expansion mainly depends on a relative increase in old subjects of CD16/CD57 double positive and CD16/CD8 dim double positive subpopulations [19]. It is not clear if this phenomenon simply represents a different distribution of NK elements among the lymphoid tissues that occurs during ageing or a true expansion of the NK compartment in the body.

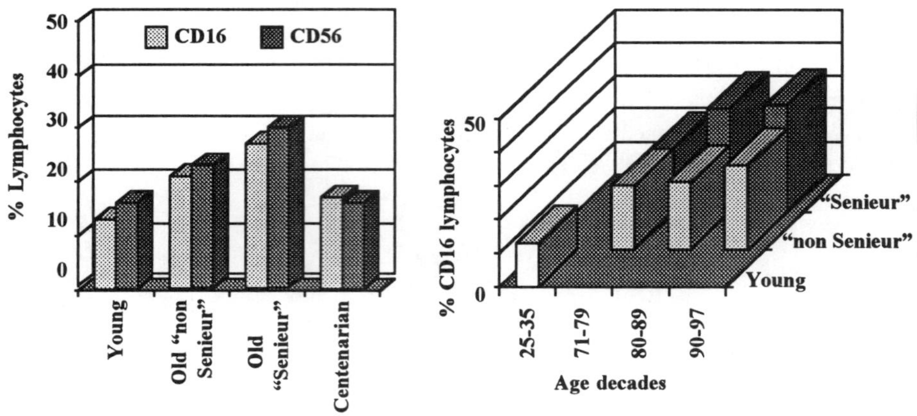

Figure 1. Phenotypical distribution of fresh unstimulated peripheral blood NK lymphocytes from young, old "Senieur", old "non-Senieur" and centenarian subjects. An increased number of NK cells (CD16, CD56) was observed in old "Senieur" ($p < 0.02$) and old "non-Senieur" ($p < 0.05$) compared to young controls. The comparative analysis of NK cells present in old and young subjects made on the basis of physical parameters did not show any difference between the mononuclear cell suspensions in the groups examined, nor in the membrane density of these molecules. When the data were analysed according to the age decades, a progressive increase in CD16 NK cells was found in "Senieur" subjects from 71 to 97 years of age ($p<0.05$ at least). Results are expressed as mean percentages of positive cells.

In a group of "non-Senieur" subjects not fulfilling all the selection criteria because of chronic respiratory infections but healthy at the time of the study, the number of CD16 cells is still elevated, but at an intermediate degree between "Senieur" and young subjects [20] (Figure 1).

In a consistent population of centenarians, representing a group undergoing a successful "natural selection", the increased number of NK cells was correlated with a reciprocal decrease of T cells in the peripheral blood ($p<0.02$), supporting our idea of a compensative increase in NK cells for a decreased cytolytic activity [21].

In agreement with these data, Remarque & Pawelec [22] demonstrated that a decrease of CD4 positive T cell numbers in very old people resulted in an increased risk of death in the elderly in the first two years after laboratory determination.

4. Spontaneous Cytolytic Activity

The cytolytic activity displayed by peripheral blood lymphocytes must be roughly dependent on the relative proportion of the NK cells present in the sample. On the contrary the cytolytic activity of NK cells, determined by evaluation of ^{51}Cr release from K562 cells following incubation with peripheral blood lymphocytes, was found to be similar in the elderly "Senieur" despite the twofold number of effector cells [16] (Figure 2). In contrast, the old "non- Senieur" group (healthy, but suffering from respiratory infections) and a population of centenarians showed a lower lytic activity than young and old " Senieur"

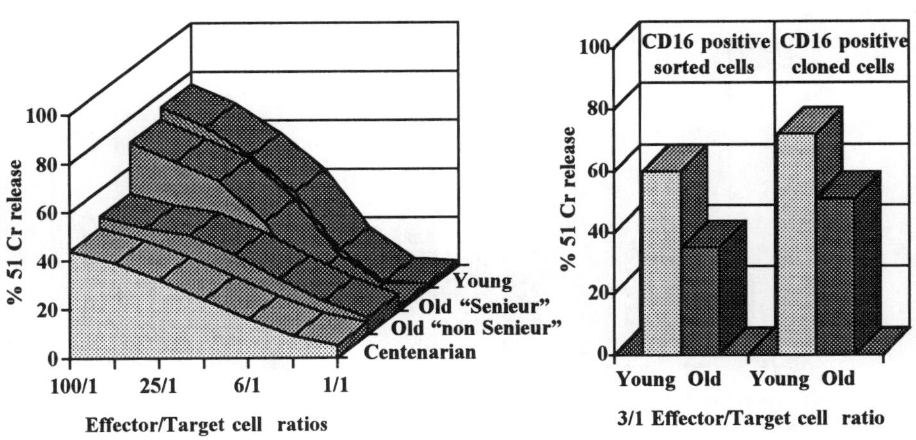

Figure 2. Cytolytic activity of peripheral blood mononuclear cells from young and old "Senieur" subjects was similar for all the effector/target cell ratios examined even though the old group presented a higher number of NK cells. Old "non-Senieur" and centenarian subjects displayed a lower activity ($p < 0.05$).
NK activity was also assayed using a pure population of CD16 cells obtained either by sorting with a FACS system or by cloning NK cell precursors. CD16 cells from old "Senieur" subjects exhibited a significantly lower cytotoxic activity ($p < 0.01$). Results are expressed as mean percentages of 51Cr release.

groups [20] (Figure 2).

In any case, when purified populations of NK cells were used to assess NK cytotoxicity, CD16-positive cells (obtained by cell sorting or after cloning procedures) showed a decreased cytolytic activity in the aged on a per cell basis [16, 23] (Figure 2).

Since cytolytic activity is the result of complex interactions between effector and target cells involving recognition and binding between the effector cell and its target, conjugate formation, lysis of target cells and recycling of the effector cell to start another cytotoxic cycle, we tried to evaluate the different steps of the reaction, analysing binding and killing using a single target/effector cell ratio.

5. Conjugate Formation and Lytic Efficiency

A similar binding capacity of single NK cells to a target tumour cell (number of conjugates between NK cells and K562 targets) was demonstrated in young and old subjects both when total lymphocytes or CD16-positive cells, electronically identified, were used [16, 19] (Figure 3).

When NK lytic efficiency (number of conjugates between CD16-positive cells and K562 cells presenting a killed K562 target) was evaluated at single cell level, by flow cytometry which allows a large number of cells to be counted, the lytic efficiency of CD16-positive cells bound to target cells from the elderly was about half that displayed by young people [19], confirming results obtained with total lymphocytes [16] (Figure 3).

These data suggest that, during ageing, the binding between NK cells and tumour targets

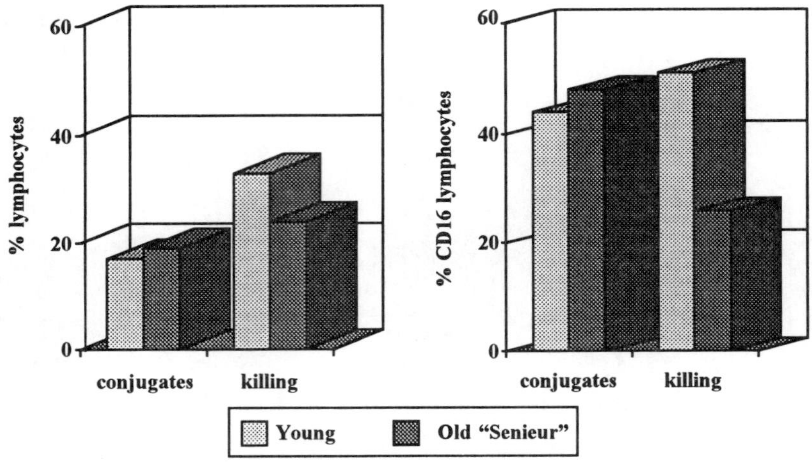

Figure 3. The ability of effector cells to bind and lyse K562 was determined at the single cell level in mononuclear cell suspensions and in CD16 lymphocytes from young and old "Senieur" subjects. The percentage of conjugates represents the percentage of mononuclear cells bound to K562 target cells to form a conjugate. The percentage of killing represents the percentage of conjugates containing a killed K562 target cell.

Target cell binding was similar in the two groups, but the ability to lyse the bound target cells appeared to be significantly less in aged subjects in comparison with the young ($p < 0.05$).

is not affected, but the multistep interaction process between the NK cell and its target is impaired after binding, probably due to a decreased activity of the lytic machinery or an inefficient transduction of the activating signal.

6. Adhesion Structures

A major role in the binding between effector cells and their targets is played by several families of adhesion receptors. In agreement with the data on binding, the expression of some of these molecules on CD16 positive cells is maintained in the elderly.

CD11a, CD11b, CD18 and CD58 molecules were expressed on the majority of CD16-positive cells in old and young alike (Figure 4), while CD2 and CD54 were in general less represented on NK cells but more in the old group than in the young and with a similar surface density [21, 24]. The enhanced expression of some of these molecules in the aged may suggest a compensation for a decreased ability of elderly NK cells to monitor the environment by contact interaction. It is also possible that NK cells from old subjects expressed more adhesion molecules on their membranes due to a continuous activation in vivo by exposure to autologous target cells. Alternatively, the level of these molecules may be upregulated due to an inefficient transduction of the activation signal.

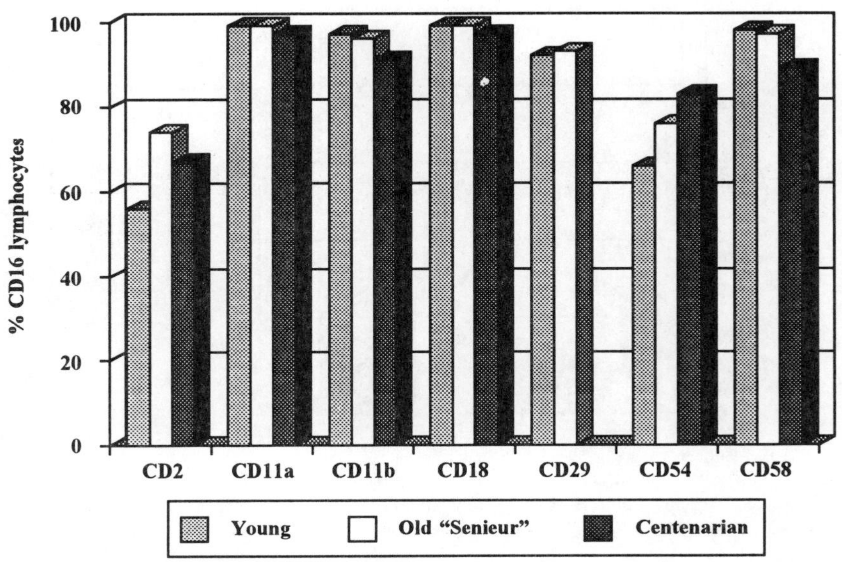

Figure 4. Expression of adhesion molecules by NK peripheral blood lymphocytes. A two colour immunofluorescence was used to characterise the expression of the various molecules, by CD16-positive populations defined by electronic gating with a FACStar Plus. CD11a, CD11b, CD18, CD29 and CD58 were expressed in more than 85% of the CD16 lymphocytes, while CD2 and CD54 were in general less represented in the CD16-positive population; they were higher in the old groups than in the young ($p < 0.02$). The results are expressed as mean percentages of positive cells.

7. Inhibitory Receptors

Surface receptors for defined MHC class I alleles expressed on NK cells are used as receptors for determinants of MHC class I molecules on target cells and this interaction delivers an inhibitory signal that prevents NK-mediated lysis of targets [25]. Different types of receptor, specific for groups of HLA-C (p58 molecules) or HLA-B alleles have been identified and are recognised by CD158a and b [26], and CD94 monoclonal antibodies respectively [27]. CD158 a, b molecules were widely distributed on NK cells of both young and old subjects and an increased number of these cells from elderly subjects were double stained [28, 29], paralleling the difference found in the peripheral blood. Also the CD94 molecule was more expressed on old NK cells (Figure 5).

Neoplastic and virally infected cells may change the expression of class I molecules, modifying the susceptibility of these cells to appropriate allele specificity; therefore a preserved ability of NK cells to recognise heterogeneous alleles is particularly important in the elderly. Together with the presence of the receptor on NK cells, its membrane-density may also be relevant for the development of an optimal negative signal after the interaction with specific HLA alleles and this parameter is also to be conserved in the elderly.

In general, people who age in good health present a pattern of HLA haplotypes for the character "lysis" similar to the general population and seem not to undergo a natural

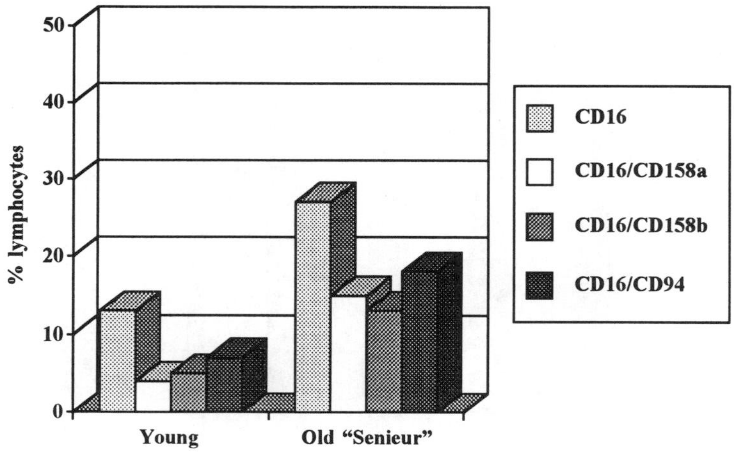

Figure 5. Distribution of CD158a, CD158b (p58 molecules) and CD94 on NK lymphocytes from young and old "Senieur" subjects. Results are expressed as mean percentages of positive cells.

selection of NK subpopulations for a particular antigen of HLA class I, at least for these molecules.

8. Lytic Mechanism

Essentially two major mechanisms by which cytotoxic lymphocytes lyse tumour target cells have been proposed: a) the "apoptotic" pathway whereby the effector-target cell interaction triggers a programmed cascade for cell death and dissolution, involving the interaction of the Fas ligand (a type II membrane protein) expressed on the effector cells and the corresponding antigen on the target; b) the other widely accepted model attributes a central role to "exocytosis" of lytic molecules from the cytoplasm granules of the effector cell that form transmembrane pores in the target cell membrane at the site of contact [30].

Although it is only a minor component of cytolytic granules, which also contain granzymes, proteases and lysosomal enzymes [31], perforin is essential at the beginning of target cell lysis [32] and purified granules and perforins have been implicated as a cytolytic effector mechanism of cell-mediated cytotoxicity [33]. Although the recognition system used by CD8 and CD16 cells differs, their effector mechanisms are very similar [34] because they contain cytoplasmic granules with cytolytic molecules.

A similar distribution of perforin in the cytoplasm of CD8-positive and CD16-positive cells was found during ageing as in the young. The number of CD8-positive peripheral lymphocytes that constitutively expressed cytoplasm perforins in young and old "non Senieur" groups accounted for 60-65%, while in the old "Senieur" subjects more CD8 lymphocytes contained perforins (about 85%) (Figure 6). Almost all CD16-positive lymphocytes contained cytoplasmic perforins; therefore these double positive cells maintained a distribution parallel to CD16 single positive cells in each group of subjects [20]

(Figure 6).

Old subjects also maintained their ability to utilize perforins in the generation of cytolytic activity. In fact, an evident depletion of perforins from cytolytic cells was observed both in CD8-positive lymphocytes and in CD16-positive cells after incubation with K562 target cells, but the decrease was more evident in CD16 cells of the old groups suggesting that these subjects used more perforin than the young to lyse K562 targets to a similar degree.

Perforin release was specifically observed only after incubation of the effector cells with the K562 NK-susceptible line, while no release was observed using the NK-resistant lines, like Daudi cells [20]. Perforin synthesis in culture following activation with PHA was unaffected by age.

These data suggest that the age-related decline in the lytic activity of NK cells cannot be attributed merely to a difference in the frequency of perforin-positive cells. We can assume that an increased utilisation of cells allows old "Senieur" donors to maintain a lytic activity similar to the young, and that a minor depletion of these cells caused a low cytolytic activity in old "non-Senieur" subjects.

The doubled number of NK cells with perforins in the old "Senieur" group can be considered a numeric compensation for a decreased lytic activity and could be the result of a positive selection for an optimal ageing of the immune system. On the contrary, in the old group with chronic recurrent infections ("non-Senieur"), the increase in CD16/perforin-positive cells is not sufficient to compensate for the decreased functional activity nor to prevent illness and may represent a manifestation of a deficiency of the senescent immune

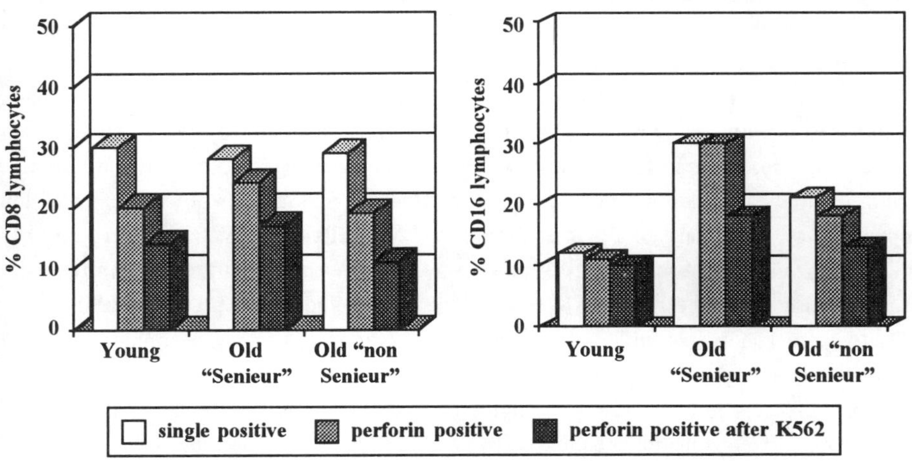

Figure 6. Perforin expression in CD8 and CD16 lymphocytes following interaction with K562 target cells. A two colour immunofluorescence was used to characterise the intracellular perforin content (identified by the G9 monoclonal antibody anti-human perforins). The cells were stained in suspension directly without previous purification or selection of a defined subset and were analysed by flow cytometry on electronically gated CD8 or CD16 cells. A depletion of perforin content in CD8 single positive cells was observed after K562 stimulation ($p < 0.05$ at least) for all the groups. CD16 single positive cells were increased in old "Senieur" ($p < 0.02$) and old "non-Senieur" ($p < 0.05$) and more than 90% contained cytoplasm perforins (CD16 perforin positive), paralleling the distribution of single positive cells. An evident decrease of CD16-positive cells was observed after K562 incubation mainly in old groups ($p < 0.05$ at least).

system. According to whether the compensatory increase in NK cells is complete or incomplete it could be related to the more ("Senieur") or less ("non-Senieur") efficient recovery from recurrent infections which could determine the development of a chronic process in old "non-Senieur" subjects. Therefore, despite a maintained distribution of perforins in cytolytic cells and a maintained or increased number of cytolytic cells producing perforins, the old subjects had a reduced lytic activity. In addition, a critical intracellular level of perforins inside cytolytic cells is required for an efficient lytic activity, only relatively few perforins are ready to be released and the remaining pool cannot be activated immediately.

We can speculate that other factors may account for the different pattern of lytic activity found in aged people. These include an altered time course or a less efficient perforin polymerisation and/or a different resynthesis speed of perforins, or a different recycling rate to kill other target cells or a defective signal transduction for granule exocytosis.

9. Signal Transduction

Recognition and binding between NK and target cells involves the stimulation of membrane receptors, the generation and transduction of signals through the cell membrane and the development of a biochemical response that determines the activation of NK cytolytic function [35]. These signalling patterns are similar to those that accompany TCR complex activation and include early phosphorylation of inositol triphosphate via phosphoinositide hydrolysis, activation of protein kinase C and a temporal elevation in the intracellular Ca^{2+} concentration [36].

We observed a pronounced age-related decrease in the ability of NK cells to generate second messengers following incubation with a similar amount of NK susceptible K562 targets. The time course formation of inositol triphosphate (IP_3) was the same as in the young with a peak approximately 15 min after stimulation, but the major biochemical defect appears to be a decrease of IP_3 formation in old NK cells (75% of the young levels) [37] (Figure 7). Since we observed an essentially preserved density of surface receptors involved in recognition and adhesion on NK cells during ageing and also a preserved ability of NK cells to form conjugates with target cells, signal transduction may be impaired at a step distal to the binding of receptors .

This defect is not associated with lower concentrations of metabolically active IP_3 precursors, (PI-phosphatidylinositol, PIP-phosphatidylinositol monophosphate or PIP_2 - phosphatidylinositol biphosphate) while it may be related to the delayed PIP_2 hydrolysis that we observed.

The ability of a target cell to trigger phosphoinositide hydrolysis in the NK effector cells depends on the degree of susceptibility of the target cell to NK cell-mediated lysis also in old subjects. In fact, we did not observe phosphoinositide hydrolysis following stimulation with non-susceptible cell lines.

NK-resistant target cells can became susceptible to NK lysis and undergo an antibody dependent cell-mediated cytotoxicity when coated with appropriate antibodies that trigger

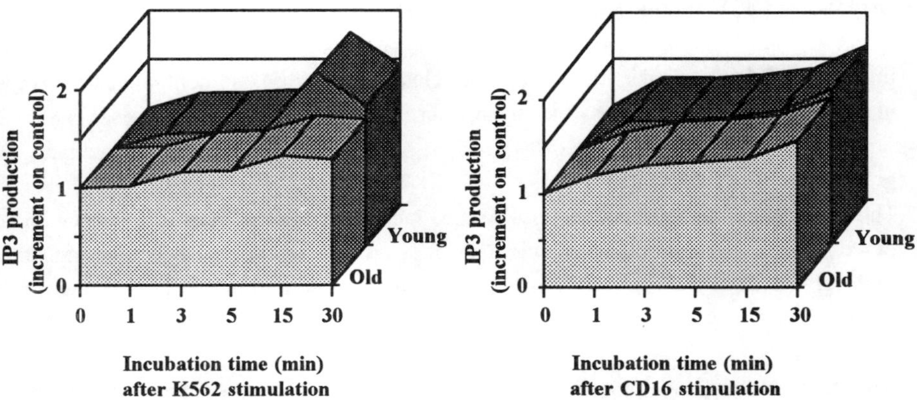

Figure 7. Inositol triphosphate (IP3) production after stimulation of purified NK cells for different time intervals. Co-incubation of human purified NK cells with a corresponding number of K562 target cells produced a progressive increase in IP3, with the peak approximately 15 min after the beginning of stimulation followed by a gradual slight decline in both groups. However, IP3 amount in old subjects was significantly reduced at 15 min when compared with the level produced by NK cells from young subjects ($p < 0.05$). Fc activation of NK cells with CD16 monoclonal antibody consistently increased IP3 levels over those present in unstimulated cells and developed almost comparable kinetics between young and old subjects. Results are expressed as increment on control unstimulated NK cells.

the Fc receptor [38]. From the beginning of Fc activation with CD16 and with almost comparable kinetics, a rapid and stable increase in IP_3 levels over those present in unstimulated cells (Figure 7) together with a concomitant hydrolysis of PIP_2 was observed in young and old subjects.

Recent studies demonstrated that distinct biochemical pathways were activated after recognition of susceptible tumour or antibody-coated targets [39]. The different phosphorylation patterns induced and the consequent differential activation varied with the nature of the ligand and the discrimination is very selective [39, 40, 41].

Changes observed in spontaneous cytolytic activity together with qualitative and quantitative differences in PIP_2 and IP_3 formation following K562 target interaction but not observed in ADCC or following Fc receptor triggering, confirm that different biochemical pathways of activation exist in NK cells also in old subjects when target or antibody-mediated activation occurs and that the selectivity of the response is preserved. Alternatively, these findings could reflect a different activation threshold for the molecules/receptors involved in cytolytic responses.

Since enhancement of natural killer cell activation induced by inositol phosphate, correlates with tumour suppression, our results may offer important insights into which NK effector functions may be differentially modulated in vivo (bypassing the defective component), to reverse or improve declines in cell-mediated immune functions associated with advancing age. In addition, it may be possible to reduce the incidence of diseases that become prevalent in later life and develop an experimental and therapeutic strategy to counteract endogenous down-regulation of NK responses.

10. Metabolism of Vitamin D, Body Mass and NK Cells

Immune endocrine and nervous systems are closely integrated and communicate through circulating cytokines, hormones and neurotransmitters [42]. Many hormones have an important influence on the homeostasis of the immune system and in maintaining the integrity of body composition [13, 14].

The age-related decrease in adipose tissue, muscle and bone mass together with an increased risk of malnutrition and vitamin deficiency are among the major factors implicated in the development of frailty syndromes in the elderly. As a consequence, these changes may induce decreased physical ability, altered energy metabolism and impaired resistance to infections.

NK cell number and cytolytic activity were significantly associated with serum concentrations of vitamin D (Figure 8) and this association was consistent with the evidence that vitamin D supplementation in elderly subjects in vivo significantly modulated NK activity, increasing circulating levels of α-IFN [21].

A poor vitamin D availability is frequently encountered in elderly people due to a reduced dietary intake, solar exposure and skin production [43]. States of vitamin D deficiency are associated with defective non-specific immune response (probably secondary to a block of the cell cycle progression due to a decreased production of cytokines involved in activation of lymphocytes) and are consistent with the presence in vivo of receptors for the hormone on cells of the immune system [44]. Age-related changes in vitamin D metabolism favour increased serum levels of iPTH which was inversely correlated with NK cell number.

Besides being involved in immune regulation, this hormonal axis is also a regulator of bone metabolism by means of various cytokines common to the two systems [45].

During normal ageing a progressive body mass erosion is described for a loss of both lean and fat mass, with a consequent reduced ability to provide energetic substrates during stress conditions [46, 47].

Anthropometric parameters indicating fat reserves (AFA-arm fat area and TST-triceps skinfold thickness) and muscle reserve (AMA-arm muscle area) were also directly correlated with NK cell number and activity and fat indicators were linked to vitamin D (Figure 8).

Immune and nutritional evaluations represent specific and sensitive prognostic indices in predicting complications in hospitalised or free-living elderly subjects, because their

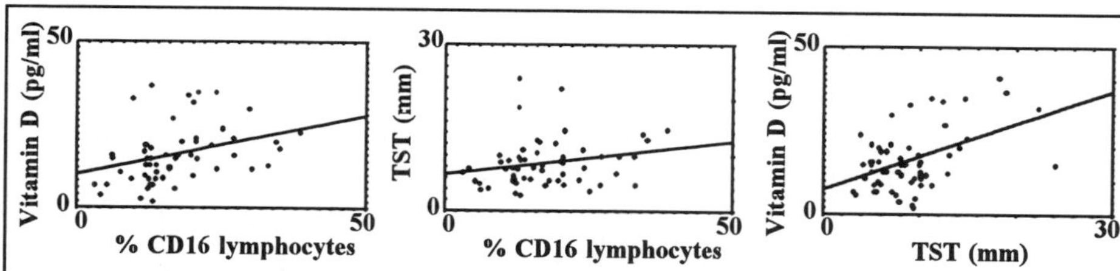

Figure 8. Scatterplot of vitamin D, TST and NK (CD16) lymphocyte number. Direct correlations were found between the increase in CD16 positive lymphocytes, vitamin D ($p<0.001$) and TST ($p<0.02$) and between the increase in vitamin D and TST ($p<0.05$).

appropriate immune response is influenced by nutritional status. It is therefore not surprising that both bone and muscle remodelling hormones and anthropometric indices of very old subjects correlated so well with their NK function, and that a similar association was found for daily living activities The physical autonomy of oldest-old people strongly depends on muscular mass strength and on calorie fat stores.

The close correlation between the degree of malnutrition and immunodeficiency in the elderly may increase the risk of infection as demonstrated by the high number of subjects unresponsive to influenza vaccination among undernourished aged subjects [48]. Catabolic conditions can have dramatic repercussions in oldest-old subjects with chronic diseases or with reduced metabolic reserve, and because of the close interrelations between malnutrition and immunodeficiency, these results stress the paramount importance of nutritional evaluation in the clinical assessment of elderly people.

Acknowledgements

It was a pleasure to meet all the researchers of the EUCAMBIS group and in particular the authors thank Prof. Graham Pawelec from Tubingen, project leader and Prof. Rafael Solana from Cordoba for the friendly team work. Many thanks also to our past students Dr. Alessandra Meneghetti and Dr. Andrea Tarozzi for the days spent on the experimental procedures, to Anne Collins for revising the English manuscript, Patrizia Rappini and Graziella Salmi for editorial assistance.
This work was performed under the aegis of the European Union Concerted Action on the Molecular Biology of Immunosenescence EUCAMBIS (contract BMHI-CT94-1209) and partially supported by grants from M.U.R.S.T. (60% fund) and from Ricerca Corrente I.O.R., University of Bologna, Italy.

References

[1] J. O'Shea and J.R. Ortaldo, The biology of natural killer cells: insights into the molecular basis of function. In: C.E. Lewis and J.O. McGee (eds.), The natural immune system. The natural killer cell. IRL Press, Oxford, 1991, pp. 2-40.

[2] H.F. Pross and E. Lotzova, Role of natural killer cells in cancer. *Nat. Immun.* **12** (1993) 209-217.

[3] J.C. Roder, T. Haliotis, M. Klein, S. Korec, J.R. Jett, J. Ortaldo, R.B. Herberman, P. Katz, and A.S. Fauci, A new immunodeficiency disorder in humans involving NK cells. *Nature* **284** (1980) 553-555.

[4] E. Grunebaum, G.E. Malatzky, and Y. Shoenfeld, Natural killer cells and autoimmunity. *Immunol. Res.* **8** (1989) 292-304.

[5] N.G. Klimas, F.R. Salvato, R. Morgan, and M.A. Fletcher, Immunologic abnormalities in chronic fatigue syndrome. *J. Clin. Microbiol.* **28** (1990) 1403-1410.

[6] M. Irwin, M. Brown, T. Patterson, R. Hauger, A. Mascovich, and I. Grant, Neuropeptide Y and natural killer cell activity: findings in depression and Alzheimer caregiver stress. *Neural Modul. Immunol.* **5** (1991) 3100-3107.

[7] L. Hoffman-Goetz and B.K. Pedersen, Exercise and the immune system: a model of the stress response? *Immunol. Today* **15** (1994) 382-387.

[8] K. Nakachi and K. Imai, Environmental and physiological influences on human natural killer cell activity in relation to good health practices. *Jpn. J. Cancer Res.* **83** (1992) 798-805.

[9] M. Irwin, C. Caldwell, T.L. Smith, S. Brown, M.A. Schuckit, and C. Gillin, Major depressive disorder, alcoholism, and reduced natural killer cell cytotoxicity. *Arch. Gen. Psychiatry* **147** (1990) 713-719.

[10] H.F. Pross and M.G. Baines, Studies of human natural killer cells. I. In vivo parameters affecting normal cytotoxic function. *Int. J. Cancer* **29** (1982) 383-390.

[11] J.S. Goodwin, Decreased immunity and increased morbidity in the elderly. *Nutrition Rev.* **53** (1995) S41-S44.

[12] G. Pawelec, M. Adibzadeh, H. Pohla, and K. Schaudt, Immunosenescence: ageing of the immune system. *Immunol. Today* **16** (1995) 420-422.

[13] B.M. Lesourd and S. Meaume, Cell mediated immunity changes in ageing, relative importance of cell subpopulation switches and of nutritional factors. *Immunol. Lett.* **40** (1994) 235-242.

[14] R. Chandra, Nutrition and immunity in the elderly: clinical significance. *Nutrition Rev.* **53** (1995) S80-S85.

[15] G.J. Ligthart, J.X. Corberand, C. Fournier, P. Galanaud, W. Hijmans, B. Kennes, H.K. Muller-Hermelink, and G.G. Steinmann, Admission criteria for immunogerontological studies in man: the SENIEUR protocol. *Mech. Ageing Dev.* **28** (1984) 47-55.

[16] A. Facchini, E. Mariani, A.R. Mariani, S. Papa, M. Vitale, and F.A. Manzoli, Increased number of circulating Leu11+ (CD16) large granular lymphocytes and decreased NK activity during human ageing. *Clin. Exp. Immunol.* **68** (1987) 340-347.

[17] G.J. Ligthart, P.C. van Vlokhoven, H.R. Schuit, and W. Hijmans, The expanded null cell compartment in ageing: increase in the number of natural killer cells and changes in T-cell and NK-cell subsets in human blood. *Immunology* **59** (1986) 353-357.

[18] R. Krishnaraj and G. Blandford, Age-associated alterations in human natural killer cells. 2. Increased frequency of selective NK subsets. *Cell. Immunol.* **114** (1988) 137-148.

[19] M. Vitale, L. Zamai, L.M. Neri, A. Galanzi, A. Facchini, R. Rana, A. Cataldi, and S. Papa, The impairment of natural killer function in the healthy aged is due to a postbinding deficient mechanism. *Cell. Immunol.* **145** (1992) 1-10.

[20] E. Mariani, S. Sgobbi, A. Meneghetti, M. Tadolini, A. Tarozzi, M. Sinoppi, L. Cattini, and A. Facchini, Perforins in human cytolytic cells: the effect of age. *Mech. Ageing Dev.* **92** (1996) 195-209.

[21] E. Mariani, G. Ravaglia, A. Meneghetti, A. Tarozzi, P. Forti, F. Maioli, F. Boschi, and A. Facchini, Natural immunity and bone and muscle remodelling hormones in the elderly. *Mech. Ageing Dev.* **102** (1998) 279-292.

[22] E. Remarque and G. Pawelec, T cell immunosenescence and its clinical relevance in man. *Rev. Clin. Gerontol.* **8** (1998) 5-25

[23] E. Mariani, P. Roda, A.R. Mariani, M. Vitale, A. Degrassi, S. Papa, and A. Facchini, Age-associated changes in CD8+ and CD16+ cell reactivity: clonal analysis. *Clin. Exp. Immunol.* **81** (1990) 479-484.

[24] E. Mariani, M.C.G. Monaco, L. Cattini, M. Sinoppi, and A. Facchini, Distribution of adhesion molecules on CD4, CD8 and CD16 lymphocytes during ageing. In: F. Licastro and C.M. Caldarera (eds.), Biomarkers of aging: expression and regulation. Editrice CLUEB, Bologna, 1992, pp. 341-348.

[25] A. Moretta, R. Biassoni, C. Bottino, D. Pende, M. Vitale, A. Poggi, M.C. Mingari, and L. Moretta, Major histocompatibility complex class I-specific receptors on human natural killer and T lymphocytes. *Immunol. Rev.* **155** (1997) 105-117.

[26] A. Moretta, C. Bottino, and R. Biassoni, CD158a (p58.1/p50.1) and CD158b (p58.2/p50.2) natural killer receptors for HLA-C alleles: workshop panel report. In: T. Kishimoto, H. Kikutani, A.E.G. Kr von dem Borne, A.M. Goyert, D.Y. Mason, M. Miyasaka, L. Moretta, K. Okumura, S. Shaw, T.A. Springer, K. Sugamura, and H. Zola (eds.), Leukocyte typing VI. Garland Publishing, Inc. New York, 1997, pp. 290-292.

[27] M. Lopez-Botet, J.J. Perez-Villar, M. Carretero, A. Rodriguez, I. Melero, T. Bellon, M. Llano, and F. Navarro, Structure and function of the CD94 C-type lectin receptor complex involved in recognition of HLA class I molecules. *Immunol. Rev.* **155** (1997) 165-174.

[28] E. Mariani, M.C.G. Monaco, L. Cattini, M. Sinoppi, and A. Facchini, Distribution and lytic activity of NK cell subsets in the elderly. *Mech. Ageing Dev.* **76** (1994) 177-187.

[29] E. Mariani, S. Sgobbi, A. Meneghetti, A. Tarozzi, L. Cattini, and A. Facchini, CD158a and b workshop: distribution of p58 molecules on peripheral blood lymphocytes during ageing. In: T. Kishimoto, H. Kikutani, A.E.G. Kr von dem Borne, A.M. Goyert, D.Y. Mason, M. Miyasaka, L. Moretta, K. Okumura, S. Shaw, T.A. Springer, K. Sugamura, and H. Zola (eds.), Leucocyte typing VI. Garland Publishing,Inc. New York, 1997, pp. 304-306.

[30] G. Berke, The binding and lysis of target cells by cytotoxic lymphocytes: molecular and cellular aspects. *Annu. Rev. Immunol.* **12** (1994) 735-773.

[31] J. Tschopp and M. Nabholz, Perforin-mediated target cell lysis by cytolytic T lymphocytes. *Annu. Rev. Immunol.* **8** (1990) 279-302.

[32] C.C. Liu, C.M. Walsh, and J.D.E. Young, Perforin: structure and function. *Immunol. Today* **16** (1995) 194-201.

[33] W.R. Clark, C.M. Walsh, A.A. Glass, F. Hayashi, M. Matloubian, and R. Ahmed, Molecular pathways of CTL-mediated cytotoxicity. *Immunol. Rev.* **146** (1995) 33-44.

[34] D. Kägi, B. Ledermann, K. Bürki, R.M. Zinkernagel, and H. Hengartner, Lymphocyte-mediated cytotoxicity in vitro and in vivo: mechanisms and significance. *Immunol. Rev.* **146** (1995) 95-115.

[35] K.P. Windebank, R.T. Abraham, G. Powis, R.A. Olsen, T.J. Barna, and P.J. Leibson, Signal transduction during human natural killer cell activation: inositol phosphate generation and regulation by cyclic amp. *J. Immunol.* **141** (1988) 3951-3957.

[36] S.G. Ward, S.C. Ley, C. MacPhee, and D.A. Cantrell, Regulation of D-3 phosphoinositides during T cell activation via the T cell antigen receptor/CD3 complex and CD2 antigens. *Eur. J. Immunol.* **22** (1992) 45-49.

[37] E. Mariani, A.R. Mariani, A. Meneghetti, A. Tarozzi, L. Cocco, and A. Facchini, Age-dependent decreases of NK cell phosphoinositide turnover during spontaneous but not Fc mediated cytolytic activity. *Int. Immunol.* **10** (1998) 981-989.

[38] T. Takai, M. Li, D. Sulvestre, R. Clynes, and J.V. Ravetch, FcR gamma chain deletion results in pleiotrophic effector cell defects. *Cell* **76** (1994) 519-529.

[39] J.D. Bonnema, L.M. Karnitz, R.A. Schoon, R.T. Abraham, and P.J. Leibson, Fc receptor stimulation of phosphatidylinositol 3-kinase in natural killer cells is associated with protein kinase C-independent granule release and cell-mediated cytotoxicity. *J. Exp. Med.* **180** (1994) 1427-1435.

[40] C.R. Yu, J.X. Lin, D.W. Fink, S. Akira, E.T. Bloom, and A. Yamauchi, Differential utilisation of Janus kinase-signal transducer activator of transcription signalling pathways in the stimulation of human natural killer cells by IL-1, IL-12, and IFN-alpha. *J. Immunol.* **157** (1996) 126-137.

[41] A. Sulica, D. Metes, M. Gherman, T.L. Whiteside, and R.B. Herberman, Divergent effects of Fc gamma RIIIA ligands on the functional activities of human natural killer cells in vitro. *Eur. J. Immunol.* **26** (1996) 1199-1203.

[42] H.O. Besedovsky and A. Del Rey, Immune-neuroendocrine circuits: integrative role of cytokines. Frontiers in Neuroendocrinology. Raven Press, New York, 1992, pp. 61-94.

[43] F. Ravaglia, P. Forti, L. Pratelli, F. Maioli, C.R. Scali, A.M. Bonini, S. Tedioli, N. Marasti, A. Pizzoferrato, and G. Gasbarrini, The association of ageing with calcium active hormone status in men. *Age Ageing* **23** (1994) 127-131.

[44] S.C. Manolagas, F.G. Hustmyer, and X.P. Yu, 1,25-Dihydroxyvitamin D3 and the immune system. *Proc. Soc. Exp. Biol. Med.* **191** (1989) 238-245.

[45] G. Weryha and J. Leclere, Paracrine regulation of bone remodelling. *Horm. Res.* **43** (1995) 69-75.

[46] G.A. Borkan and A.H. Norris, Fat redistribution and the changing body dimensions of the adult male. *Human Biol.* **49** (1977) 495-514.

[47] R. Roubenoff and J.J. Kehayias, The meaning and measurement of Lean Body Mass. *Nutrition Rev.* **49** (1991) 163-175.

[48] B.M. Lesourd, Protein undernutrition as the major cause of decreased immune function in the elderly: clinical and functional implications. *Nutrition Rev.* **53** (1995) S86-S91.

EUCAMBIS: Immunology and Ageing in Europe
G. Pawelec (Ed.)
IOS Press, 2000

Phenotypic and functional analysis of NK cells in the elderly

Corona Alonso, Francisco Borrego, Belén Ostos, José Peña, Rafael Solana.
Department of Immunology. (rsolana@uco.es), Faculty of Medicine. "Reina Sofia" University Hospital. University of Córdoba. Spain.

Abstract. Although the process of immunosenescence affects mainly to T cells, age-associated alterations in natural killer (NK) cell phenotype and function have also been demonstrated. It has been shown that NK cell cytotoxicity is well preserved in healthy elderly people fulfilling Senieur criteria and also in healthy octogenarians and even in centenarians. A significant expansion in the number of NK cells expressing a mature phenotype is also found in aging. Antibody-dependent cellular cytotoxicity (ADCC) remains comparable between young and elderly subjects. However, NK cell killing of K562 is impaired when considered on a per cell basis. This defect is associated with defective PKC-coupled transmission signals as a consequence of aging. Furthermore, the response to IL2 is impaired when proliferation, expression of CD69 and cytotoxicity of NK-resistant cell lines are considered, but not when K562 killing is considered. Aging does not alter other NK cell functions such as perforin content and lymphokine production (TNF-α). These results support the hypothesis that aging significantly affect NK cell phenotype and function, although the effect of senescence is different, depending on the NK cell functions considered.

1. Introduction

The term immunosenescence refers to the significant decline in the immune response found in aged persons and animals. Although the T cell compartment of the immune system is the most affected by aging, complex age-associated immunological alterations occur in other cells of the immune system in elderly people [1-3], including the innate immunity and natural killer (NK) cells [4;5]. Human NK cells represent a heterogeneous lympnoid population involved in the recognition and lysis of tumor and virally infected cells and defined by the $CD3^-$, $CD16^+$ (FcγRIIIA), $CD56^+$ (N-CAM) surface phenotype, that do not rearrange immunoglobulin (Ig) or T-cell receptor (TCR) genes and that do not express neither surface Ig nor the TCR/CD3 complex, except for the ζ chain [6-9].

The most characteristic marker of human NK cells is CD56, although in the last few years, a number of receptors, mainly expressed on NK cells and therefore considered to being NK differentiation antigens, have been identified. CD56 is an isoform of the neural cell adhesion molecule (N-CAM) and it is virtually identical to the 140 kD isoform expressed in the nervous system [10]. The precise function of CD56 in NK cells is still poorly understood although it has been suggested that CD56 is involved in homophilic adhesion between NK cells and human CD56+ tumor cell lines [11]. Another NK marker, CD57 is an oligosaccharide antigenic determinant associated with a variety of polypeptides that have not been characterized in detail. CD57 can be found on a subpopulation (approx. 50%) of NK cells and in a minor population of T lymphocytes [8;10;12]. CD16, the 50-65 transmembrane form of the IgG Fc receptor (FcRgamma III) is also a human NK cell-associated antigen. It is also expressed on macrophages and granulocytes and plays a central role in the activation of NK cells [13-17]. CD94, a C-lectin type invariant glycoprotein that associates with NKG2 products, is another NK cell differentiation antigen that is broadly expressed on NK cells although it may appear undetectable in a subset of fresh peripheral blood NK cells [8;18-20].

Accumulated evidence in the last few years has clearly established that NK cell cytotoxicity results from a balance between activating and inhibitory signals delivered by specific membrane receptors (Figure 1) [21-24]. Thus, it has been shown that NK cells express receptors that inhibit killing of potential target cells. These inhibitory receptors are specific for polymorphic MHC class I molecules and inhibit killing of target cells bearing the appropriate class I allotypes. Two distinct families of genes encoding receptors for polymorphic MHC class I molecules have been defined. The first includes inhibitory receptors encoded by multiple genes encoding type I transmembrane molecules and belonging to the immunoglobulin superfamily that have recently been localized on human chromosome 19q13.4. These include a family of genes coding for killer immunoglobulin-like receptors (KIR) expressed on NK cells and on a minor subset of T-lymphocytes, and immunoglobulin-like transcripts (ILT-1, - 2 and 3) expressed on myeloid cells and subsets of lymphoid cells. These receptors have one to four extracellular immunoglobulin domains. The KIR family of receptors includes CD158a, CD158b, p70 (NKB1) and p140 receptors for HLA-A, B and C alleles [25-30]. These inhibitory receptors are responsible of conferring NK cells the capacity to interact with specific aminoacid sequences (positions 77-84) in the α-helix of the HLA class I molecules [31-35]. In the ILT superfamily ILT2 or LIR inhibitory receptors specific for HLA-G and the cytomegalovirus protein UL18 can be included [36-38]. The second family of NK receptors encodes C-type lectin heterodimers composed of CD94 covalently associated with NKG2A, [19;39-41] which recognizes HLA-E molecules associated with peptides derived from the leader sequence of other HLA antigens [42-45]. These killer cell inhibitory receptors, that block not only natural killing, but also CD16 or CD69 triggered cytotoxicity, possess immunoreceptor tyrosine-based inhibitory motifs (ITIM) in the cytoplasmic domains that recruit the SH2-containing protein tyrosine phosphatases, SHP-1 and SHP-2, resulting in inhibition of NK cell-mediated cytotoxicity and cytokine secretion [46-50].

In relationship to the activation of NK cell cytotoxicity, no "major" NK receptor has been defined. On the contrary several molecules capable of triggering NK cytotoxicity of target cells have been defined. Although the best-characterized activatory receptor is CD16, other molecules, such as CD2, p46 [51], CD69 [50;52;53], NKRP1 [54], NKp44 [55] and the activatory HLA specific receptors p50 [56-58] and CD94/NKG2C [19;59;60], can also be involved in the activation of NK cytolysis.

CD16 (Fc gamma RIII) is a hetero-oligomeric receptor composed of a ligand-binding alpha subunit associated with homo- or heterodimers of the TCRζ- and FcεRIγ-chains. The activatory signals triggered by CD16 crosslinking involve the phosphorylation of the zeta and gamma chain coupled to the receptor. CD16 engagement in human NK cells induces rapid association of the tyrosine- phosphorylated receptor complex with the adapter protein shc. Engagement of CD16 induces the tyrosine phosphorylation of other substrates, including the phospholipase C γ-1 and γ-2 isoforms, ZAP-70 and also a rapid tyrosine phosphorylation of Cbl, which is constitutively associated with Grb2 and forms an activation-dependent complex with the p85 subunit of Pl-3K [13-17;61;62]. CD2 signal transduction in NK cells also depends upon the ζ subunit activation of the CD16 complex [63;64]. Another NK-specific triggering surface molecule that has been recently shown to

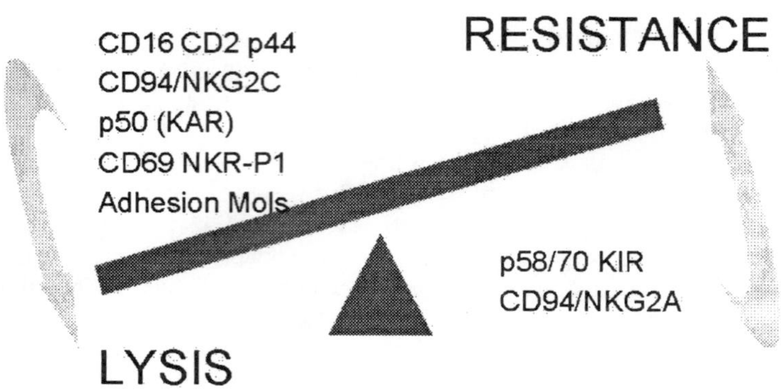

Figure 1.- Human NK lysis. Killing of target cells depends of a balance between activation and inhibition signals triggered by NK receptors.

be involved in the process of NK cell activation, p46, is also coupled to the ζ signal transduction pathway [51].

As stated above NK cells express receptors specific for polymorphic MHC class I alleles. These MHC specific receptors were first described as inhibitory receptors that block NK cytotoxicity after interaction with the appropriate HLA antigen on the target surface. However, it was found that highly homologous receptors, differing mainly in the intracellular domain, could also function as NK activatory receptors, able to trigger NK cytotoxicity in different experimental models. It has been recently described that the activatory counterparts of the HLA specific inhibitory killer receptors p50 (KIRD2S) and CD94/NKG2C are found to be non-covalently associated with the molecule DAP12, a disulfide-bonded homodimer containing an immunoreceptor tyrosine-based activating motif (ITAM) in its cytoplasmic domain [60;65]. Phosphorylated DAP12 peptides bind ZAP-70 and Syk protein tyrosine kinases, suggesting that the activation pathway is similar to that of the T- and B-cell antigen receptors [60] . Crosslinking of these receptors results in cellular activation, as demonstrated by tyrosine phosphorylation of cellular proteins and upregulation of early- activation antigens [60]. The DAP12 signal transduction activation pathway is also coupled to a novel 44-kD surface molecule, (NKp44), selectively expressed on IL-2 activated NK cells and capable of mediating strong triggering of NK cell cytotoxicity in a redirected killing assay [55].

2. Effect of aging on NK cell cytotoxicity.

Immunosenescence primarily affects the T cell compartment of the immune system, but age-associated immunological alterations also occur in NK cell phenotype and function [1-3]. NK cells play an important role in natural surveillance against viral infections and neoplastic diseases. Since non-MHC restricted killing of target cells is the most characteristic function of NK cells, the cytotoxic capacity of NK cells has been extensively analyzed in elderly people. Although originally these reports showed that NK cell activity of peripheral blood lymphocytes was not significantly affected by aging, more recent studies have demonstrated age associated changes in the number and function of NK cells [5;66].

Thus it is generally accepted that NK cytotoxicity of total peripheral blood lymphocytes is not significantly affected in aging when the studies were performed using NK cells obtained from healthy elderly people [67-72]. However, our and others' quantitative analysis of NK cells (Figure 2) show that the number of cells expressing NK cell markers is significantly increased in aged people, when compared to young or middle aged groups [5;66;73;74].

The increased number of CD56+ cells is mainly due to the expansion of the $CD56^{dim}$ subset. The level of expression of CD56 antigen defines two subpopulations of NK cells that differ in phenotype and function [75;76]. The first, defined by the low expression of CD56 ($CD56^{dim}$), comprises 90-95% of total NK cells and displays an intense cytotoxic activity. Conversely, the second group is defined by the high surface expression of CD56 ($CD56^{bright}$) and exhibits a negligible ability to lyse target cells but strongly proliferate in response to IL2 [76]. The analysis of these subpopulations in human elderly shows a decrease in the percentage of $CD56^{bright}$ in the group of elderly people when compared to the young group. However, neither the absolute number of $CD56^{bright}$ cells nor the expression of other phenotypic markers (CD25, CD94 or HLA-DR) in this subpopulation are significantly affected in senescence [66]. These results indicate that the increased percentage of NK cells observed in the elderly is the consequence of the expansion of the $CD56^{dim}$ subset more than a defective production of $CD56^{bright}$ cells. Our results support previous observations that suggested a phenotypic and functional shift to the maturity status of NK cells in aging [77]. The results indicating that the increase in the number of peripheral NK cells did not correlate with a significant increase in the cytotoxic activity of these cells, suggested that NK cell cytotoxicity should be impaired when considered in a per cell basis [73]. Mariani et al [78] have shown that circulating NK cells from elderly subjects have a decreased cytotoxic function both after sorting freshly isolated cells and after limiting dilution and cloning of NK cell precursors. Furthermore it has also

Figure 2.- Expression of T and NK cell markers in elderly and young healthy donors (adapted from ref. 66).

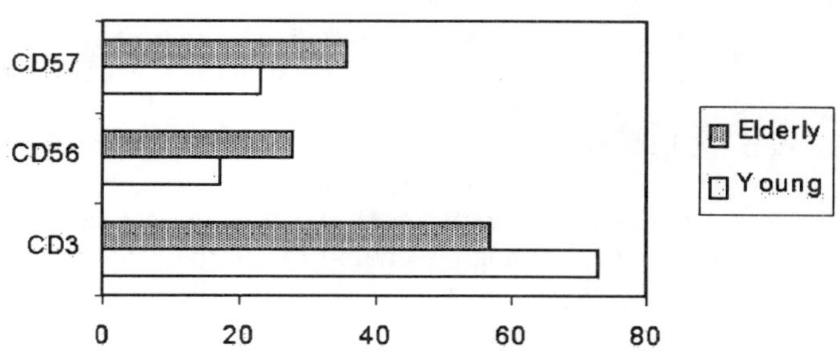

been shown that the defective NK cell cytotoxicity is associated to a decreased capacity of NK cells to release IP3 after interacting with the target cells and a delayed hydrolysis of PIP2, indicating that the PKC dependent pathway is affected as a consequence of aging [79].

NK cells also mediate cytotoxicity when triggered by the Fc receptor (CD16). Thus the CD16:ζ:γ receptor complex allows natural killer (NK) cells to recognize and eliminate antibody-coated target cells. This process, termed antibody-dependent cellular cytotoxicity (ADCC), has also been studied in the peripheral blood lymphocytes of aging subjects. The results from different authors have shown that ADCC was comparable between young and aging subjects [80-83]. Furthermore the PI-3-kinase pathway triggered by CD16 crosslinking is not significantly affected in NK cells from elderly people, indicating that aging differentially affects the transduction pathways involved in natural or CD16-dependent NK cytotoxicity [79]. Recent studies, using a flow cytometric technique, have shown suggested that the deficiency in the cytolytic activity could be related with an age-related decrease both in the percentage of NK cells expressing perforin and in the mean levels of perforin per cell [84]. However, other authors have not demonstrated a diminished perforin content or to a defect in the granule redistribution on NK cells from aged individuals [85], suggesting that the signal transduction defect are the main responsible of the defective cytotoxicity observed in NK cells from elderly healthy individuals.

The role of NK cells in the defense against infectious diseases in the elderly has been recently underscored. Thus Ogata et al., [86] have found decreased NK cell activity in a group of 44 healthy elderly individuals. Furthermore, they also studied whether any of the immunologic parameters determined, including lymphocyte subsets counts and NK cell cytotoxicity, was related to past infectious episodes and death in the follow-up period. The results obtained demonstrated that low NK cell cytotoxicity, considered either as absolute values or on a per-cell basis, was the only parameter that correlated with a past history of severe infection or death due to infection in the elderly group.

3. NK cells from elderly people have a decreased response to IL2.

In addition to cytotoxicity NK cells also have other functions, such as proliferation or cytokine production in response to IL-2. We have studied whether these non-cytotoxic functions of NK cells are affected by aging. The results show that purified NK cells from healthy Senieur donors have a significantly decreased proliferative capacity when compared to the young group. [66]. A significant decrease in the expression of CD69 induced by IL2 was also observed (Figure 3). However, there is a broad variation in the response from quasi-normal to a virtually absent proliferation. These differences did not correlate with age or sex. They did not correlate with clinical conditions either, as all individuals in the group fulfilled the Senieur criteria of healthy aging. The proliferative response in each individual parallels the expression of CD69 antigen induced by IL-2 activation, indicating that the defective proliferation is due to a general defect in the NK cell response to IL-2. This deterioration in NK cell response that occurs in aging is pronounced in some aged individuals, subtle in others and even negligible in some.

In addition, the increase in the cytolytic activity of NK cells in response to several cytokines has also been studied [68;69]. Treatment of NK cells with different cytokines

Figure 3.-CD69 expression and proliferative response of purified NK cells obtained from Senieur elderly and young controls after IL-2 stimulation (adapted from ref. 66).

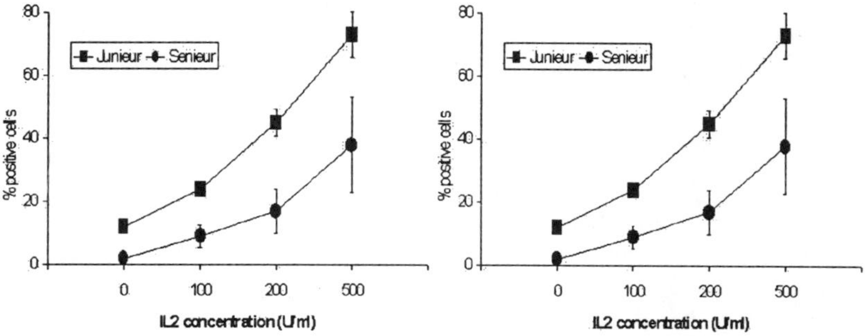

augments NK cell cytotoxicity against both NK sensitive and NK resistant cell lines. NK treatment with IL-2, IL-12 or IFN-α enhances cytotoxicity of the NK sensitive target K562 in both young and elderly samples. The same degree of increase was observed over a wide range of doses and incubation times. However, the cytotoxic capacity of these cytokine activated killer cells against the normally NK-resistant Daudi cell line was significantly decreased in the elderly when compared to young people [68;69].

Therefore, these results suggest that NK cells have an age-associated defect in their response to cytokines with a subsequent decreased capacity to develop LAK cells able to kill NK resistant cell lines. Other authors have shown that cytokine (IL-2 and interferon alpha and gamma) induced anti-tumor MHC-unrestricted cytotoxic activity of NK cells is well preserved in the healthy elderly [87;88]. Although the discrepancies in the results can be the consequence of the selection criteria of healthy elderly individuals, a factor that must not be underestimated in these studies, other aspects, such as experimental differences among the research groups, have to be considered. In this sense the type of cells used as targets may have a particular relevance because NK cells can use different mechanisms to kill different targets. The differential susceptibility of target cells to perforin, TNF or fas mediated cytolysis may result in differences in NK cell killing after cytokine stimulation.

4. NK cytotoxicity in centenarians

Centenarians are the best example of successful aging, since they have escaped the major age-associated diseases. As shown in healthy Senieur donors, NK cell cytotoxicity is well preserved in this population, whereas other compartment of the immune response, in particular T cell proliferation and lymphokine production, are strongly impaired [89-91]. The number and function of NK cells in this group of "very old" people, has been recently studied in relation to their basal metabolism, life style and nutritional status. Cluster analysis, used to explore the relationships among these variables, demonstrated the existence of two composed clusters linked to NK cell number, cytolytic activity and vitamin D level [92]. Thus, those individuals with higher NK cell numbers and cytolytic activity levels have better ability to develop an autonomous life style, higher serum vitamin D levels, are well-nourished subjects and have a balanced basal metabolism. It has been shown that vitamin D treatment restores impaired NK cell activity in haemodyalisis patients [93] supporting a role for this hormone in the regulation of NK cell function in aging.

5. Cytokine production by NK cell from elderly donors.

To further investigate the effect of aging in other non-cytotoxic functions of NK cells we have also studied the secretion of TNF-α in response to IL-2. Our results show that TNF-α production by purified NK cells from elderly people is not significantly affected when compared to young donors [66]. However it has been reported that the amount of IFN-γ secreted by purified, 18 h activated NK cells from the elderly was only 25 percent of that released by the cells from the young. This aging-related early phase secretory deficit could be overcome by culturing NK cells for 7 days with rIL-2 [94].

The profile of cytokine production by different cell populations is broadly altered in senescence. Leukocytes of the elderly produced higher amounts of IL-1, IL-6, IL-8 and TNF-α after induction with lipopolysaccharide (LPS) than leukocytes from young donors. In contrast, in vitro induction of IFN-α by viruses is decreased in the elderly compared to the young. In a similar way the production of the TH1 cytokine, IFN-γ, by unfractionated peripheral blood lymphocytes of the elderly is decreased, whereas the TH2 cytokines IL-4 and IL-10 are produced in greater amounts as compared to young individuals. The production of proinflammatory cytokines such as IL- 1, IL-6, IL-8, and TNF-α is increased in the elderly [95].

6. NK cell subsets in elderly people.

A significant expansion of NK cells, mainly due to an increase in the $CD56^{dim}$ subset, can be found in the elderly. However, this is not the only phenotypic change associated with NK cells in aging. Analysis of the activation markers on NK cells demonstrates that their expression is significantly affected in the $CD56^{dim}$ subset. Thus, the expression of HLA-DR and CD95 is significantly increased in NK cells from Senieur donors, while the expression of CD69 is decreased compared to its expression in NK cells from young donors [66]. These results indicate that, although overall MHC unrestricted cytotoxicity seems normal in elderly people, changes in the phenotype and in other NK cell functions can be detected. The definition in the last few years of new NK-associated receptors has made it necessary to analyze if their expression is altered in old people. Despite the better knowledge and understanding of NK receptors involved in the regulation of NK cell cytotoxicity, very little is known of the possible involvement of any of these receptors in the defective individual NK cell function found in the elderly. It has been shown that the expression of killer inhibitory receptors (p58) is not significantly affected in NK cells from elderly donors when compared with NK cells from young controls [96]. However, the functional relevance of these findings is difficult to evaluate since the mAbs used in these studies react with extracellular epitopes present in both the inhibitory and activatory forms of the KIR2D receptor (anti-p58 EB6, GL183 and HP3E4 also recognize the p50 activatory counterparts).

7. T cell expression of NK differentiation markers in aging.

Aged mice expressed elevated percentages of NK1.1+ T cells in their secondary lymphoid organs, peripheral blood and liver [97;98]. These murine NK1.1+ T cells are extrathymic T cells, produce IL-4 and their central role in the anti-tumor cytotoxic response triggered by IL12 has been recently defined [99-102]. It has been suggested that the minor subpopulation of human T cells that also express NK markers (i.e., CD56, CD57) might be the human counterpart of the NK1.1+ T cells found in mice. The origin and function of this human minor T cell subpopulation is still poorly understood, although it has been suggested that they are generated extrathymically [103]. An expansion of this T cell subset has been demonstrated in patients with colorectal carcinoma [103] and in knee joints and adjacent bone marrow of rheumatoid arthritis patients [104]. Increased expression of CD94 in NK and T cells from HIV-1 infected individuals has also been shown [105]. We have also found (Figure 4) a significant increase in the expression of the NK differentiation antigens CD57 and CD94 on T cells in the elderly [66]. A significant increase with age has also been found both in the absolute counts and in the proportions of CD3 positive T cells that co-express CD16/CD56 antigens, whereas the $CD57^{+}CD8^{high}$ subset, which represent the cytolytic T cell population, showed less change with age [106]. Increased proportions of $CD3^{+}CD56^{+}$ T and $CD3^{+}CD57^{+}$ T cells have also been found in centenarians [107]. These results suggest that there is a major shift in lymphocyte population from conventional T cells to NK cells and extrathymic T cells with senescence.

Figure 4.- Co-expression of NK cell markers on T cells from elderly and young healthy donors. Values are referred to total number of CD3 or CD56 cells (adapted from ref. 66).

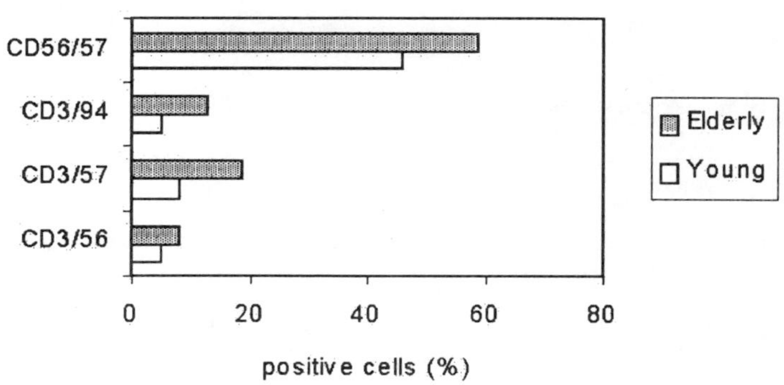

8. Concluding remarks

The deterioration of the immune system associated with aging defined as immunosenescence is characterized by a decreased T cell response to antigens although changes in the humoral response and in the number and function of other cells of the immune system can also be observed. Thus, age-associated alterations have been demonstrated in NK cell phenotype and function. The NK cytotoxic capacity of total peripheral blood lymphocytes is well preserved not only in healthy elderly people but also in centenarians. The maintenance of NK cell cytotoxicity is associated with a significant expansion in the number of NK cells expressing a mature phenotype. Therefore NK cell killing of K562 is impaired when considered in a per cell basis and this defect is associated to defective PKC-coupled transmission signals as a consequence of aging. Furthermore, the response to IL2 is impaired when proliferation, expression of CD69 and cytotoxicity of NK-resistant cell lines are considered, but not when K562 killing is considered. Aging does not alter other NK cell functions such as perforin content and lymphokine production (TNF-α). These results suggest that human NK cells do not escape the aging process, and that senescence has a differential effect on distinct NK cell biological functions, ranging from severe to negligible impairment, depending on the parameters considered. Recent evidence suggests that a low NK cell function relates to the development of severe infections in elderly subjects and indicates that well preserved NK cell cytotoxicity is a parameter clinically relevant for survival, presumably by protecting aged individuals against infectious disease. More studies on the possible changes in the inhibitory and stimulatory receptors that control NK cell cytotoxicity during aging are required to better understand the process of NK cell immunosenescence. Furthermore, the effect of T cell senescence in the regulation of NK cell cytotoxicity, the effect of the changes observed in the cytokine network on NK cell differentiation and activation as well as the mechanisms involved in NK cell signal transduction require further investigation.

Acknowledgements: This work was supported by grants from Fondo Investigación Sanitaria (FIS95/1242, FIS 98/1052) and Junta de Andalucía (Spain) and was carried out under the aegis of the European Union Concerted Action on the Molecular Biology of Immunosenescence (EUCAMBIS; Biomed I contract CT94-1209).

References

1 G. Pawelec and R. Solana, Immunosenescence. *Immunol Today*, **18** (1997) 514-516.

2 G. Pawelec, E. Remarque, Y. Barnett and R. Solana, T cells and aging. *Front Biosci.*, **3** (1998) d59-d99.

3 G. Pawelec, M. Adibzadeh, R. Solana and I. Beckman, The T cell in the ageing individual. *Mech Ageing Dev*, **93** (1997) 35-45.

4 G. Pawelec, R. Solana, E. Remarque and E. Mariani, Impact of aging on innate immunity. *J Leukoc Biol*, **64** (1998) 703-712.

5 R. Solana, M.C. Alonso and J. Pena, Natural killer cells in healthy ageing. *Exp Gerontol*, **(in press)** (1999)

6 G. Trinchieri, Biology of natural killer cells. *Adv Immunol*, **47** (1989) 187-376.

7 G. Trinchieri, Definition and biology of natural killer cells. In: R. Solana and J. Pena (eds.), MHC antigens and NK cells. ISBN: 1-57059-062-1. R.G. Landes Co., Austin TX, 1994, pp. 1-15.

8 M.J. Robertson and R. Solana, Reactivity and functional properties of NK-cell panel mAb. In: S.F. Schlossman, et al. (eds.), Leucocyte Typing V. ISBN: 0 19 2623761. Oxford University Press, Oxford, New York, Tokio, 1995, pp. 1373-1374.

9 R. Solana and J. Pena, Natural Killer cells receptors: activation and inhibition of NK cell mediated cytotoxicity. In: R. Solana and J. Pena (eds.), MHC antigens and NK cells. ISBN: 1-57059-062-1. R.G. Landes Co., Austin TX, 1994, pp. 16-34.

10 L.L. Lanier and J.J. Hemperly, CD56 and CD57 cluster workshop report. In: S.F. Schlossman, et al. (eds.), Leucocyte Typing V. ISBN: 0 19 2623761. Oxford University Press, Oxford, New York, Tokio, 1995, pp. 1398-1400.

11 T. Nitta, H. Yagita, K. Sato and K. Okumura, Involvement of CD56 (NKH-1/Leu-19 antigen) as an adhesion molecule in natural killer-target cell interaction. *J Exp Med*, **170** (1989) 1757-1761.

12 F. Borrego, M.D. Galiani, J.A. Madueno, L. Perez-Bermejo, F. Garcia-Cozar, J. Pena and R. Solana, Phenotypic and functional characterization of NK mAb using resting NK cells and the NK-cell line YT . In: S.F. Schlossman, et al. (eds.), Leucocyte Typing V. ISBN: 0 19 2623761. Oxford University Press, Oxford, New York, Tokio, 1995, pp. 1373-1374.

13 L.L. Lanier, G. Yu and J.H. Phillips, Co-association of CD3 zeta with a receptor (CD16) for IgG Fc on human natural killer cells. *Nature*, **342** (1989) 803-805.

14 P. Anderson, M. Caligiuri, C. O'Brien, T. Manley, J. Ritz and S.F. Schlossman, Fc gamma receptor type III (CD16) is included in the zeta NK receptor complex expressed by human natural killer cells. *Proc Natl Acad Sci U S A*, **87** (1990) 2274-2278.

15 P. Moingeon, C.C. Stebbins, L. D'Adamio, J. Lucich and E.L. Reinherz, Human natural killer cells and mature T lymphocytes express identical CD3 zeta subunits as defined by cDNA cloning and sequence analysis. *Eur J Immunol*, **20** (1990) 1741-1745.

16 E. Vivier, P. Morin, C. O'Brien, B. Druker, S.F. Schlossman and P. Anderson, Tyrosine phosphorylation of the Fc gamma RIII(CD16): zeta complex in human natural killer cells. Induction by antibody-dependent cytotoxicity but not by natural killing. *J Immunol*, **146** (1991) 206-210.

17 J.J. O'Shea, A.M. Weissman, I.C. Kennedy and J.R. Ortaldo, Engagement of the natural killer cell IgG Fc receptor results in tyrosine phosphorylation of the zeta chain. *Proc Natl Acad Sci U S A*, **88** (1991) 350-354.

18 M. Lopez-Botet, CD94 cluster report: overview of the characterization of the Kp43 NK-cell-associated surface antigen. In: S.F. Schlossman, et al. (eds.), Leucocyte Typing V. ISBN: 0 19 2623761. Oxford University Press, Oxford, New York, Tokio, 1995, pp. 1437-1439.

19 M. Lopez-Botet, J.J. Perez-Villar, M. Carretero, A. Rodriguez, I. Melero, T. Bellon, M. Llano and F. Navarro, Structure and function of the CD94 C-type lectin receptor complex involved in recognition of HLA class I molecules. *Immunol Rev*, **155** (1997) 165-174.

20 M. Lopez-Botet, M. Carretero, T. Bellon, J.J. Perez-Villar, M. Llano and F. Navarro, The CD94/NKG2 C-type lectin receptor complex. *Curr Top Microbiol Immunol*, **230** (1998) 41-52.

21 L. Moretta, E. Ciccone, A. Poggi, M.C. Mingari and A. Moretta, Ontogeny, MHC class I specificity and receptors of human natural killer cells. In: R. Solana and J. Pena (eds.), MHC antigens and NK cells. ISBN: 1-57059-062-1. R.G. Landes Co., Austin TX, 1994, pp. 92-104.

22 J. Pena and R. Solana, Effect of target cell histocompatibility antigens in NK-cell mediated recognition and lysis. In: R. Solana and J. Pena (eds.), MHC antigens and NK cells. ISBN: 1-57059-062-1. R.G. Landes Co., Austin TX, 1994, pp. 16-34.

23 M. Lopez-Botet, L. Moretta and J. Strominger, NK-cell receptors and recognition of MHC class I molecules. *Immunol Today*, **17** (1996) 212-214.

24 L.L. Lanier, NK cell receptors. *Annu Rev Immunol*, **16** (1998) 359-393.

25 A. Moretta and L. Moretta, HLA class I specific inhibitory receptors. *Curr Opin Immunol*, **9** (1997) 694-701.

26 A. Moretta, R. Biassoni, C. Bottino, D. Pende, M. Vitale, A. Poggi, M.C. Mingari and L. Moretta, Major histocompatibility complex class I-specific receptors on human natural killer and T lymphocytes. *Immunol Rev*, **155** (1997) 105-117.

27 A. Moretta, C. Bottino, M. Vitale, D. Pende, R. Biassoni, M.C. Mingari and L. Moretta, Receptors for HLA class-I molecules in human natural killer cells. *Annu Rev Immunol*, **14** (1996) 619-648.

28 E.O. Long and N. Wagtmann, Natural killer cell receptors. *Curr Opin Immunol*, **9** (1997) 344-350.

29 M. Colonna, Natural killer cell receptors specific for MHC class I molecules. *Curr Opin Immunol*, **8** (1996) 101-107.

30 L.L. Lanier, B. Corliss and J.H. Phillips, Arousal and inhibition of human NK cells. *Immunol Rev*, **155** (1997) 145-154.

31 M. Colonna, G. Borsellino, M. Falco, G.B. Ferrara and J.L. Strominger, HLA-C is the inhibitory ligand that determines dominant resistance to lysis by NK1- and NK2-specific natural killer cells. *Proc Natl Acad Sci U S A*, **90** (1993) 12000-12004.

32 J.E. Gumperz, V. Litwin, J.H. Phillips, L.L. Lanier and P. Parham, The Bw4 public epitope of HLA-B molecules confers reactivity with natural killer cell clones that express NKB1, a putative HLA receptor. *J Exp Med*, **181** (1995) 1133-1144.

33 R. Biassoni, M. Falco, A. Cambiaggi, P. Costa, S. Verdiani, D. Pende, R. Conte, C. di Donato, P. Parham and L. Moretta, Amino acid substitutions can influence the natural killer (NK)-mediated recognition of HLA-C molecules. Role of serine-77 and lysine-80 in the target cell protection from lysis mediated by "group 2" or "group 1" NK clones. *J Exp Med*, **182** (1995) 605-609.

34 I. Luque, R. Solana, M.D. Galiani, R. Gonzalez, F. Garcia, d.C.J. Lopez and J. Pena, Threonine 80 on HLA-B27 confers protection against lysis by a group of natural killer clones. *Eur J Immunol*, **26** (1996) 1974-1977.

35 R. Biassoni, A. Pessino, A. Malaspina, C. Cantoni, C. Bottino, S. Sivori, L. Moretta and A. Moretta, Role of amino acid position 70 in the binding affinity of p50.1 and p58.1 receptors for HLA-Cw4 molecules. *Eur J Immunol*, **27** (1997) 3095-3099.

36 M. Colonna and J. Samaridis, Cloning of immunoglobulin-superfamily members associated with HLA-C and HLA-B recognition by human natural killer cells. *Science*, **268** (1995) 405-408.

37 D. Cosman, N. Fanger, L. Borges, M. Kubin, W. Chin, L. Peterson and M.L. Hsu, A novel immunoglobulin superfamily receptor for cellular and viral MHC class I molecules. *Immunity*, **7** (1997) 273-282.

38 M. Colonna, F. Navarro, T. Bellon, M. Llano, P. Garcia, J. Samaridis, L. Angman, M. Cella and M. Lopez-Botet, A common inhibitory receptor for major histocompatibility complex class I molecules on human lymphoid and myelomonocytic cells. *J Exp Med*, **186** (1997) 1809-1818.

39 A.G. Brooks, P.E. Posch, C.J. Scorzelli, F. Borrego and J.E. Coligan, NKG2A complexed with CD94 defines a novel inhibitory natural killer cell receptor. *J Exp Med*, **185** (1997) 795-800.

40 M. Carretero, C. Cantoni, T. Bellon, C. Bottino, R. Biassoni, A. Rodriguez, J.J. Perez-Villar, L. Moretta, A. Moretta and M. Lopez-Botet, The CD94 and NKG2-A C-type lectins covalently assemble to form a natural killer cell inhibitory receptor for HLA class I molecules. *Eur J Immunol*, **27** (1997) 563-567.

41 S. Lazetic, C. Chang, J.P. Houchins, L.L. Lanier and J.H. Phillips, Human natural killer cell receptors involved in MHC class I recognition are disulfide-linked heterodimers of CD94 and NKG2 subunits. *J Immunol*, **157** (1996) 4741-4745.

42 F. Borrego, M. Ulbrecht, E.H. Weiss, J.E. Coligan and A.G. Brooks, Recognition of Human Histocompatibility Leukocyte Antigen (HLA)-E Complexed with HLA Class I Signal Sequence-derived Peptides by CD94/NKG2 Confers Protection from Natural Killer Cell-mediated Lysis. *J Exp Med*, **187** (1998) 813-818.

43 V.M. Braud, D.S. Allan, C.A. O'Callaghan, K. Soderstrom, A. D'Andrea, G.S. Ogg, S. Lazetic, N.T. Young, J.I. Bell, J.H. Phillips, L.L. Lanier and A.J. McMichael, HLA-E binds to natural killer cell receptors CD94/NKG2A, B and C. *Nature*, **391** (1998) 795-799.

44 M. Carretero, G. Palmieri, M. Llano, V. Tullio, A. Santoni, D.E. Geraghty and M. Lopez-Botet, Specific engagement of the CD94/NKG2-A killer inhibitory receptor by the HLA-E class Ib molecule induces SHP-1 phosphatase recruitment to tyrosine-phosphorylated NKG2-A: evidence for receptor function in heterologous transfectants. *Eur J Immunol*, **28** (1998) 1280-1291.

45 N. Lee, M. Llano, M. Carretero, A. Ishitani, F. Navarro, M. Lopez-Botet and D.E. Geraghty, HLA-E is a major ligand for the natural killer inhibitory receptor CD94/NKG2A. *Proc Natl Acad Sci U S A*, **95** (1998) 5199-5204.

46 B.A. Binstadt, K.M. Brumbaugh, C.J. Dick, A.M. Scharenberg, B.L. Williams, M. Colonna, L.L. Lanier, J.P. Kinet, R.T. Abraham and P.J. Leibson, Sequential involvement of Lck and SHP-1 with MHC-recognizing receptors on NK cells inhibits FcR-initiated tyrosine kinase activation. *Immunity*, **5** (1996) 629-638.

47 D.N. Burshtyn, A.M. Scharenberg, N. Wagtmann, S. Rajagopalan, K. Berrada, T. Yi, J.P. Kinet and E.O. Long, Recruitment of tyrosine phosphatase HCP by the killer cell inhibitor receptor. *Immunity*, **4** (1996) 77-85.

48 N.M. Valiante, J.H. Phillips, L.L. Lanier and P. Parham, Killer cell inhibitory receptor recognition of human leukocyte antigen (HLA) class I blocks formation of a pp36/PLC-gamma signaling complex in human natural killer (NK) cells. *J Exp Med 1996.Dec.1.*, **184** (1996) 2243-2250.

49 L. Olcese, P. Lang, F. Vely, A. Cambiaggi, D. Marguet, M. Blery, K.L. Hippen, R. Biassoni, A. Moretta, L. Moretta, J.C. Cambier and E. Vivier, Human and mouse killer-cell inhibitory receptors recruit PTP1C and PTP1D protein tyrosine phosphatases. *J Immunol*, **156** (1996) 4531-4534.

50 F. Borrego, M.J. Robertson, J. Ritz, J. Pena and R. Solana, CD69 is a stimulatory receptor for natural killer cell and its cytotoxic effect is blocked by CD94 inhibitory receptor. *Immunology*, (in press) (1999)

51 S. Sivori, M. Vitale, L. Morelli, L. Sanseverino, R. Augugliaro, C. Bottino, L. Moretta and A. Moretta, p46, a novel natural killer cell-specific surface molecule that mediates cell activation. *J Exp Med*, **186** (1997) 1129-1136.

52 A. Moretta, A. Poggi, D. Pende, G. Tripodi, A.M. Orengo, N. Pella, R. Augugliaro, C. Bottino, E. Ciccone and L. Moretta, CD69-mediated pathway of lymphocyte activation: anti-CD69 monoclonal antibodies trigger the cytolytic activity of different lymphoid effector cells with the exception of cytolytic T lymphocytes expressing T cell receptor alpha/beta. *J Exp Med*, **174** (1991) 1393-1398.

53 F. Borrego, J. Pena and R. Solana, Regulation of CD69 expression on human natural killer cells: differential involvement of protein kinase C and protein tyrosine kinases. *Eur J Immunol*, **23** (1993) 1039-1043.

54 L.L. Lanier, C. Chang and J.H. Phillips, Human NKR-P1A. A disulfide-linked homodimer of the C-type lectin superfamily expressed by a subset of NK and T lymphocytes. *J Immunol*, **153** (1994) 2417-2428.

55 M. Vitale, C. Bottino, S. Sivori, L. Sanseverino, R. Castriconi, E. Marcenaro, R. Augugliaro, L. Moretta and A. Moretta, NKp44, a novel triggering surface molecule specifically expressed by activated natural killer cells, is involved in non-major histocompatibility complex-restricted tumor cell lysis [In Process Citation]. *J Exp Med*, **187** (1998) 2065-2072.

56 C. Bottino, S. Sivori, M. Vitale, C. Cantoni, M. Falco, D. Pende, L. Morelli, R. Augugliaro, G. Semenzato, R. Biassoni, L. Moretta and A. Moretta, A novel surface molecule homologous to the p58/p50 family of receptors is selectively expressed on a subset of human natural killer cells and induces both triggering of cell functions and proliferation. *Eur J Immunol*, **26** (1996) 1816-1824.

57 R. Biassoni, C. Cantoni, M. Falco, S. Verdiani, C. Bottino, M. Vitale, R. Conte, A. Poggi, A. Moretta and L. Moretta, The human leukocyte antigen (HLA)-C-specific "activatory" or "inhibitory" natural killer cell receptors display highly homologous extracellular domains but differ in their transmembrane and intracytoplasmic portions. *J Exp Med*, **183** (1996) 645-650.

58 A. Moretta, S. Sivori, M. Vitale, D. Pende, L. Morelli, R. Augugliaro, C. Bottino and L. Moretta, Existence of both inhibitory (p58) and activatory (p50) receptors for HLA-C molecules in human natural killer cells. *J Exp Med*, **182** (1995) 875-884.

59 K.M. Brumbaugh, J.J. Perez-Villar, C.J. Dick, R.A. Schoon, M. Lopez-Botet and P.J. Leibson, Clonotypic differences in signaling from CD94 (kp43) on NK cells lead to divergent cellular responses. *J Immunol*, **157** (1996) 2804-2812.

60 L.L. Lanier, B. Corliss, J. Wu and J.H. Phillips, Association of DAP12 with Activating CD94/NKG2C NK Cell Receptors. *Immunity*, **8** (1998) 693-701.

61 R. Galandrini, G. Palmieri, R. Paolini, M. Piccoli, L. Frati and A. Santoni, Selective binding of shc-SH2 domain to tyrosine-phosphorylated zeta but not gamma-chain upon CD16 ligation on human NK cells. *J Immunol*, **159** (1997) 3767-3773.

62 C. Cerboni, A. Gismondi, G. Palmieri, M. Piccoli, L. Frati and A. Santoni, CD16-mediated activation of phosphatidylinositol-3 kinase (PI-3K) in human NK cells involves tyrosine phosphorylation of Cbl and its association with Grb2, Shc, pp36 and p85 PI-3K subunit. *Eur J Immunol*, **28** (1998) 1005-1015.

63 E. Vivier, P.M. Morin, C. O'Brien, S.F. Schlossman and P. Anderson, CD2 is functionally linked to the zeta-natural killer receptor complex. *Eur J Immunol*, **21** (1991) 1077-1080.

64 P. Moingeon, J.L. Lucich, D.J. McConkey, F. Letourneur, B. Malissen, J. Kochan, H.C. Chang, H.R. Rodewald and E.L. Reinherz, CD3 zeta dependence of the CD2 pathway of activation in T lymphocytes and natural killer cells. *Proc Natl Acad Sci U S A*, **89** (1992) 1492-1496.

65 K.S. Campbell, M. Cella, M. Carretero, M. Lopez-Botet and M. Colonna, Signaling through human killer cell activating receptors triggers tyrosine phosphorylation of an associated protein complex. *Eur J Immunol*, **28** (1998) 599-609.

66 F. Borrego, C. Alonso, M. Galiani, J. Carracedo, R. Ramirez, B. Ostos, J. Pena and R. Solana, NK phenotypic markers and IL2 response in NK cells from elderly people. *Exp Gerontol*, (in press) (1999)

67 P. Sansoni, A. Cossarizza, V. Brianti, F. Fagnoni, G. Snelli, D. Monti, A. Marcato, G. Passeri, C. Ortolani, E. Forti and a. et, Lymphocyte subsets and natural killer cell activity in healthy old people and centenarians. *Blood*, **82** (1993) 2767-2773.

68 J. Kutza and D.M. Murasko, Effects of aging on natural killer cell activity and activation by interleukin-2 and IFN-alpha. *Cell Immunol*, **155** (1994) 195-204.

69 J. Kutza and D.M. Murasko, Age-associated decline in IL-2 and IL-12 induction of LAK cell activity of human PBMC samples. *Mech Ageing Dev*, **90** (1996) 209-222.

70 E. Sugiyama, M. Ito, H. Suzuki, N. Yamashita, M. Maruyama and S. Yano, Natural killer cell activity associated with aging and sex in humans. *Jpn J Med*, **22** (1983) 195-199.

71 M. Onsrud, Age dependent changes in some human lymphocyte sub-populations. Changes in natural killer cell activity. *Acta Pathol Microbiol Scand [C]*, **89** (1981) 55-62.

72 J.E. Ales-Martinez, M. Alvarez-Mon, F. Merino, F. Bonilla, C. Martinez, A. Durantez and A. De la Hera, Decreased TcR-CD3+ T cell numbers in healthy aged humans. Evidence that T cell defects are masked by a reciprocal increase of TcR-CD3- CD2+ natural killer cells. *Eur J Immunol*, **18** (1988) 1827-1830.

73 A. Facchini, E. Mariani, A.R. Mariani, S. Papa, M. Vitale and F.A. Manzoli, Increased number of circulating Leu 11+ (CD 16) large granular lymphocytes and decreased NK activity during human ageing. *Clin Exp Immunol*, **68** (1987) 340-347.

74 M. Vitale, L. Zamai, L.M. Neri, A. Galanzi, A. Facchini, R. Rana, A. Cataldi and S. Papa, The impairment of natural killer function in the healthy aged is due to a postbinding deficient mechanism. *Cell Immunol*, **145** (1992) 1-10.

75 M.A. Caligiuri, A. Zmuidzinas, T.J. Manley, K. Smith and Ritz.J., Functional consequences of interleukin-2 receptor expression on resting human lymphocytes. Identification of a novel natural killer cell subset with high affinitty receptors. *J Exp Med*, **171** (1990) 1509-1515.

76 D.M. Baume, M.J. Robertson, H. Levine, T.J. Manley, P.W. Schow and J. Ritz, Differential responses to interleukin 2 define functionally distinct subsets of human natural killer cells. *Eur J Immunol*, **22** (1992) 1-6.

77 R. Krishnaraj and A. Svanborg, Preferential accumulation of mature NK cells during human immunosenescence. *J Cell Biochem*, **50** (1992) 386-391.

78 E. Mariani, P. Roda, A.R. Mariani, M. Vitale, A. Degrassi, S. Papa and A. Facchini, Age-associated changes in CD8+ and CD16+ cell reactivity: clonal analysis. *Clin Exp Immunol*, **81** (1990) 479-484.

79 E. Mariani, A.R. Mariani, A. Meneghetti, A. Tarozzi, L. Cocco and A. Facchini, Age-dependent decreases of NK cell phosphoinisitide turnover during spontaneous but not Fc mediated cytotlytic activity. *Int Immunol*, **10** (1998) 981-989.

80 G. Fernandes and S. Gupta, Natural killing and antibody-dependent cytotoxicity by lymphocyte subpopulations in young and aging humans. *J Clin Immunol*, **1** (1981) 141-148.

81 D.L. Edwards and F.P. Avis, Antibody-dependent cellular cytotoxicity effector cell capability among normal individuals. *J Immunol*, **123** (1979) 1887-1893.

82 N.B. Marcano, A. Rivas, E.F. Figarella, I. Blanca, G.K. Penchaszadeh, G. Perez-Rojas and N.E. Bianco, Cell-mediated effector mechanisms in aging humans. *Int Arch Allergy Appl Immunol*, **69** (1982) 7-11.

83 G. Batory, M. Benczur, M. Varga, T. Garam, C. Onody and G.G. Petranyi, Increased killer cell activity in aged humans. *Immunobiology*, **158** (1981) 393-402.

84 D. Rukavina, G. Laskarin, G. Rubesa, N. Strbo, I. Bedenicki, D. Manestar, M. Glavas, S.E. Christmas and E.R. Podack, Age-related decline of perforin expression in human cytotoxic T lymphocytes and natural killer cells. *Blood*, **92** (1998) 2410-2420.

85 E. Mariani, S. Sgobbi, A. Meneghetti, M. Tadolini, A. Tarozzi, M. Sinoppi, L. Cattini and A. Facchini, Perforins in human cytolytic cells: the effect of age. *Mech Ageing Dev*, **92** (1996) 195-209.

86 K. Ogata, N. Yokose, H. Tamura, E. An, K. Nakamura, K. Dan and T. Nomura, Natural killer cells in the late decades of human life. *Clin Immunol Immunopathol*, **84** (1997) 269-275.

87 R. Krishnaraj, Immunosenescence of human NK cells: effects on tumor target recognition, lethal hit and interferon sensitivity. *Immunol Lett*, **34** (1992) 79-84.

88 R. Krishnaraj, Senescence and cytokines modulate the NK cell expression. *Mech Ageing Dev*, **96** (1997) 89-101.

89 P. Sansoni, A. Cossarizza, V. Brianti, F. Fagnoni, G. Snelli, D. Monti, A. Marcato, G. Passeri, C. Ortolani, E. Forti and a. et, Lymphocyte subsets and natural killer cell activity in healthy old people and centenarians [see comments]. *Blood*, **82** (1993) 2767-2773.

90 C. Franceschi, D. Monti, P. Sansoni and A. Cossarizza, The immunology of exceptional individuals: the lesson of centenarians [see comments]. *Immunol Today*, **16** (1995) 12-16.

91 A. Cossarizza, C. Ortolani, D. Monti and C. Franceschi, Cytometric analysis of immunosenescence. *Cytometry*, **27** (1997) 297-313.

92 E. Mariani, G. Ravaglia, A. Meneghetti, A. Tarozzi, P. Forti, F. Maioli, F. Boschi and A. Facchini, Natural immunity and bone and muscle remodelling hormones in the ageing. *Mech Ageing Dev*, **102** (1998) 279-292.

93 Quesada J.M., R. Solana, I. Serrano, V. Barrio, M.E. Martinez, M. Santamaria and A. Martin-Malo, Immunologic effects of vitamin D. *N Engl.J Med*, **321** (1989) 833-834.

94 R. Krishnaraj and T. Bhooma, Cytokine sensitivity of human NK cells during immunosenescence. 2. IL2- induced interferon gamma secretion. *Immunol Lett*, **50** (1996) 59-63.

95 L. Rink, I. Cakman and H. Kirchner, Altered cytokine production in the elderly. *Mech Ageing Dev*, **102** (1998) 199-210.

96 E. Mariani, M.C. Monaco, L. Cattini, M. Sinoppi and A. Facchini, Distribution and lytic activity of NK cell subsets in the elderly. *Mech Ageing Dev*, **76** (1994) 177-187.

97 M.E. Poynter, H.H. Mu, X.P. Chen and R.A. Daynes, Activation of NK1.1+ T cells in vitro and their possible role in age-associated changes in inducible IL-4 production. *Cell Immunol*, **179** (1997) 22-29.

98 A. Tsukahara, S. Seki, T. Iiai, T. Moroda, H. Watanabe, S. Suzuki, T. Tada, H. Hiraide, K. Hatakeyama and T. Abo, Mouse liver T cells: their change with aging and in comparison with peripheral T cells. *Hepatology*, **26** (1997) 301-309.

99 S. Koyasu, CD3+CD16+NK1.1+B220+ large granular lymphocytes arise from both alpha- beta TCR+CD4-CD8- and gamma-delta TCR+CD4-CD8- cells. *J Exp Med*, **179** (1994) 1957-1972.

100 J. Cui, T. Shin, T. Kawano, H. Sato, E. Kondo, I. Toura, Y. Kaneko, H. Koseki, M. Kanno and M. Taniguchi, Requirement for Valpha14 NKT cells in IL-12-mediated rejection of tumors. *Science*, **278** (1997) 1623-1626.

101 N. Arase, H. Arase, S.Y. Park, H. Ohno, C. Ra and T. Saito, Association with FcRgamma is essential for activation signal through NKR-P1 (CD161) in natural killer (NK) cells and NK1.1+ T cells. *J Exp Med*, **186** (1997) 1957-1963.

102 K. Tamada, M. Harada, K. Abe, T. Li, H. Tada, Y. Onoe and K. Nomoto, Immunosuppressive activity of cloned natural killer (NK1.1+) T cells established from murine tumor-infiltrating lymphocytes. *J Immunol*, **158** (1997) 4846-4854.

103 T. Okada, T. Iiai, Y. Kawachi, T. Moroda, Y. Takii, K. Hatakeyama and T. Abo, Origin of CD57+ T cells which increase at tumour sites in patients with colorectal cancer. *Clin Exp Immunol*, **102** (1995) 159-166.

104 K. Arai, S. Yamamura, S. Seki, T. Hanyu, H.E. Takahashi and T. Abo, Increase of CD57+ T cells in knee joints and adjacent bone marrow of rheumatoid arthritis (RA) patients: implication for an anti- inflammatory role. *Clin Exp Immunol*, **111** (1998) 345-352.

105 M.D. Galiani, E. Aguado, R. Tarazona, P. Romero, I. Molina, M. Santamaria, R. Solana and J. Pena, Expression of Killer inhibitory receptors on cytotoxic cells from HIV1 infected individuals. *Clin Exp Immunol*, in press (1998)

106 S.E. McNerlan, I.M. Rea, H.D. Alexander and T.C. Morris, Changes in natural killer cells, the CD57CD8 subset, and related cytokines in healthy aging. *J Clin Immunol*, **18** (1998) 31-38.

107 C. Miyaji, H. Watanabe, M. Minagawa, H. Toma, T. Kawamura, Y. Nohara, H. Nozaki, Y. Sato and T. Abo, Numerical and functional characteristics of lymphocyte subsets in centenarians. *J Clin Immunol*, **17** (1997) 420-429.

Author Index